MASSAGE FOR SPORT

MASSAGE
for Sport

JOAN WATT

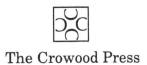

The Crowood Press

First published in 1999 by
The Crowood Press Ltd
Ramsbury, Marlborough
Wiltshire SN8 2HR

British Library Cataloguing-in-Publication Data
A catalogue record for this book is available from the British Library.

ISBN 1 86126 160 8

Acknowledgements
The author wishes to express her thanks to: Neill Watt for all his support, encouragement and help; Fiona Morrison for encouragement and final proof reading; all the athletes who have allowed her to develop her massage skills; the students who have questioned and required answers to support the practical application of massage in sport; finally to Margaret Hollis for asking her to contribute to *Massage for Therapists* and thus sparking an interest in writing.

Photo Credits
The author would like to express her thanks to Jim Mailer of Whyler Photos for all of the photography and to Jamie Morrison for acting as model.

Dedication
To the men in my life, Neill and Stewart.

Typefaces used: Galliard and Franklin Gothic.

Typeset and designed by
D & N Publishing
Membury Business Park, Lambourn Woodlands
Hungerford, Berkshire.

Printed and bound in Great Britain by
J W Arrowsmith Ltd, Bristol.

Contents

Introduction

HISTORY OF MASSAGE

The derivation of the word 'massage' is from the Greek word *massein*, meaning to knead. Massage is an age-old process that involves stimulation of the tissues by rhythmically applying both stretching and pressure.

Massage has been used in sport from time immemorial. 'Athletes have resorted to massage since the days of the first Olympic Games, and the ancient athletes developed a special tool, the strygil, to scrape the masseur's oil from the skin' (Williams, 1974). The art of massage is well documented in different countries, and skills from the East have brought many of the methods that are lauded today.

The sports public throughout the ages from the original Greeks onwards has used massage in one form or another. There are many variations and distinct differences from country to country. For example, in Great Britain the basic massage taught tends to have its origins in Swedish massage. The Chartered Society of Physiotherapists originated from a body of practitioners who first practised massage. They then added Swedish exercises and finally electrotherapy to their repertoire.

With the passage of time, massage in all its forms has largely passed out of the hands of the medical professional, and today there is a plethora of training courses and qualifications available in all massage disciplines. Sports massage is no different and with time more and more techniques have been added to the practice, some of which are more inclined towards passive exercise than massage.

The sportsperson looks for the practitioner who will give them the type of massage they want. Sadly, damage can result through lack of knowledge by both practitioner and athlete. Only recently has there been any worthwhile research into actual benefits or damage from sports massage. Statistics from the GB Athletic Team's international competitions from 1986 onwards, show that there has been no decrease in the number of massages given. Important differences are that prior to 1972 the G.B. Athletics team was as likely to have a 'physiotherapist/bag person' travel with them as a chartered physiotherapist. As treatments evolved the physio became a chartered practitioner who was as good at providing the latest electrical wizardry as giving a good massage. With the passage of time less and less massage was taught to chartered physiotherapists, so in 1990 for the first time ever the G.B. Athletics team took both chartered physiotherapists and a sports masseur with it to the European Championships in Split.

Sports massage is still evolving. It is hoped that the next chapter in its history will include the formation of a national register of suitably qualified sports masseurs with their own professional governing body and regulations, as presently happens elsewhere in the world.

CHAPTER 1
Preparation

SELF-PREPARATION OF THE SPORTS MASSEUR

As there is to be close contact and touch, it is important that the masseur takes time to prepare him or herself for the massage to be administered.

Clothing

Clothes should be loose enough to allow free, unrestricted movement while also looking neat and professional. Materials which launder easily are preferable as it is not unusual for contact with massage mediums to stain clothing. In the clinical setting, medical-style tops with trousers for both males and females are the chosen option. At the sharp end of sport the clothing used will depend very much on the setting where the massage is to be performed. In a sports hall, changing room or dedicated room it may well be that a pair of jogging trousers, tracksuit bottoms with a cotton tee-shirt or polo shirt will be best dress. If the massage is to take place in the open, for example at the track or pitch side with no overhead cover, the ambient temperature will dictate the clothing. Although the ideal top would have short sleeves, in the outdoor situation the masseur's comfort must be observed, and it may be necessary to put on a long-sleeved top either because of cold or to afford protection from the sun or rain.

Personal Hygiene

Hair should not be allowed to come into contact with the participant. If hair is long enough to touch the collar it must be tied back.

Jewellery, watches, bracelets and necklaces which may dangle over or touch the client and rings must all be removed, the exception being a narrow wedding band provided it does not cause irritation. Long/large earrings must also be removed. (Tip – have a safety pin inside the trouser pocket and put rings on this before starting a massage.)

Nails must be short, not showing above the pad of the finger and with no ragged edges or nail polish.

Hands need to be well cared for. It is essential to cleanse hands before and after each massage, and always clean hands after massaging the feet, especially if proceeding to massage another body area. In the clinical indoor situation there should be a wash hand-basin in the room where the massage is being performed. Air dryers or disposable towels are preferable to terry towelling, in order to prevent any infection spreading. At the pitch/track side moisturized tissues are the best hand cleaners (Tip – remember to have a small rubbish bag in which to place all used tissues.)

Well-cared-for hands with smooth skin are essential for the masseur. It may be necessary to prepare hands by using appropriate hand creams regularly, and especially in cold conditions a good-quality protective moisturizer is recommended. Cuts/abrasions on the hands may preclude massage being administered, unless they can be covered without the protective covering intruding onto the palmar aspect of the hand. Some practitioners wear very light rubber gloves. Hands also need to be exercised to increase their range of movement and to strengthen them. There also needs to be a good range of movement in the elbows and flexibility in the forearms.

Table 1 Hand, Arm Exercises

1. Make both hands into a fist, hold clenched for five seconds, then open out and spread fingers and thumbs as far apart as possible (Figs 1 & 2).

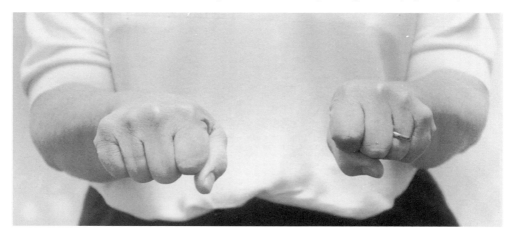

Fig 1. Exercise hand into clenched fist.

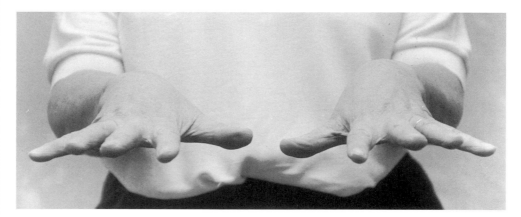

Fig 2. Spread fingers and thumb.

Table 1 Hand, Arm Exercises *(continued)*

2. Place the fingertips of one hand in contact with fingertips of other and press so that thumbs and little fingers are as widely spaced as possible (Fig 3).

3. Push two, three and finally four fingers between two adjacent fingers of the other hand to increase range of movement. Repeat in each space and for both hands (Fig 4).

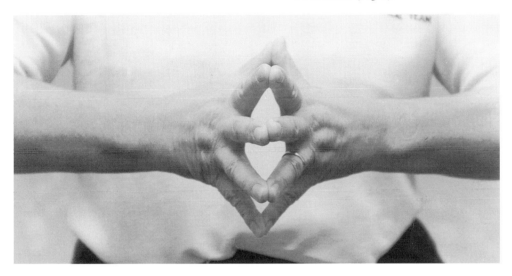

Fig 3. Exercise to increase finger and thumb span.

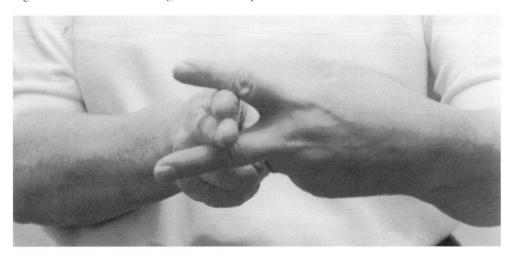

Fig 4. Exercise to increase finger span.

Table 1 Hand, Arm Exercises *(continued)*

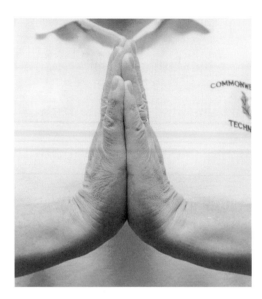

Fig 5. Start position for exercise for wrist mobility.

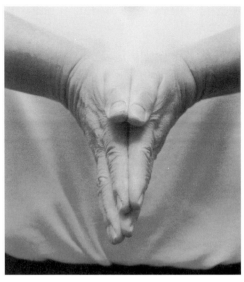

Fig 6. Finish position for exercise for wrist mobility.

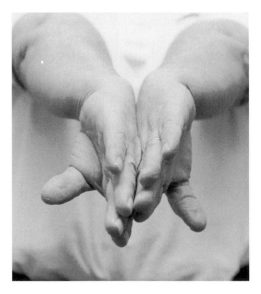

Fig 7. Start position for exercise to increase wrist flexion.

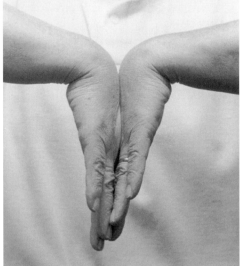

Fig 8. Finish position for exercise to increase wrist flexion.

Table 1 Hand, Arm Exercises *(continued)*

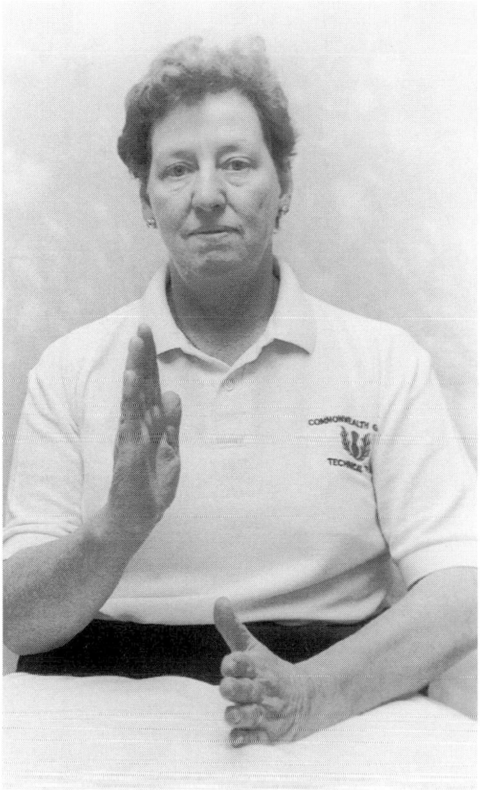

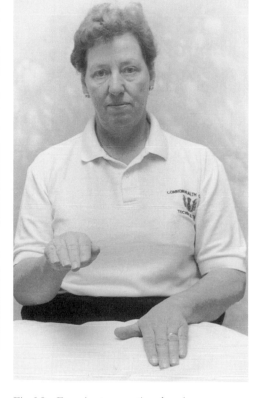

Fig 9. Practise full range pronation and supination.

Fig 10. Exercise to practise clapping.

4. Place palms of hands together, with fingers and thumbs in contact, elbows bent at chest level. Slowly turn hands to ground until fingers point down, reverse to starting position (Figs 5 & 6).

5. Place backs of hands together, with arms out straight, bend elbow up towards chin to flex wrists (Figs 7 & 8).

6. Place a pillow on your knee, start with the border of your fourth finger and hand in contact with the pillow, raise your right hand up until your thumb touches your chest and lower to start position. Repeat with left hand and alternate hand to hand until the hands are passing each other at the middle of the movemen (Fig 9).

7. Repeat exercise 6, starting with cupped hands in contact with the pillow instead of the border (Fig 10).

Table 1 Hand, Arm Exercises *(continued)*

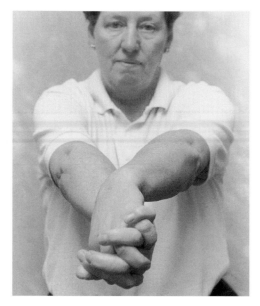

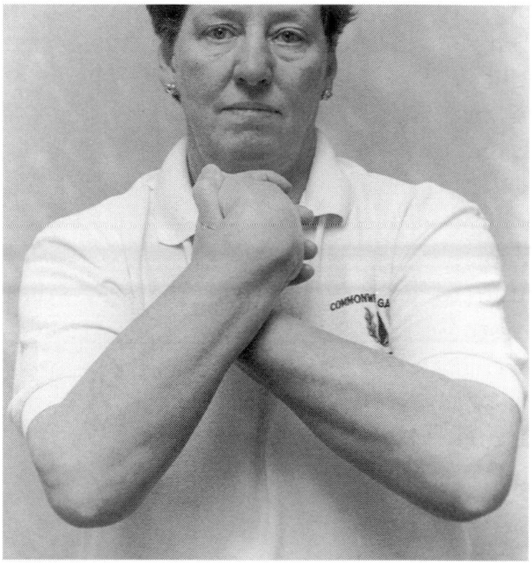

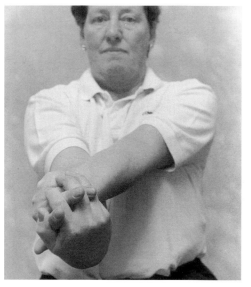

Fig 11. *(Above)* Start position for exercise to increase wrist and forearm mobility.

Fig 12. *(Above left)* Mid position for exercise to increase wrist and forearm mobility.

Fig 13. *(Right)* Finish position for exercise to increase wrist and forearm mobility.

8. Clasp hands with wrists crossed, elbows straight, bend elbows to bring hands up to chin, straighten elbows out, keeping hands firmly clasped at all times. Do not force. Go only as far as is possible (Figs 11, 12 & 13).

Stance

Massage can be very time-consuming and it is vitally important that the masseur does not end up being exhausted.

Optimum Posture

If you are standing with your left side next to the client, your right leg should be in front, with the knee slightly bent. Practise this stance with your arms stretched out and transfer your weight from front leg to back leg (Fig 14). Also practise standing with your front to the client, again with one knee bent and arms stretched out, then transfer your weight forward and backwards (Fig 15).

In the clinical situation there should be a massage couch available but at pitch/track side this will not always be the case and you will have to improvise and use whatever is available. Try to avoid having to kneel on the ground to perform massage, as this is not comfortable for either the recipient or practitioner. Make use of stand seating, exercise mats, pole vault or high jump landing beds or changing room seating. **Remember at all times to protect your back and not put your optimum posture at risk**.

Relaxation

It is important that the hands and forearms are relaxed to allow full hand contact with the body part that is to be massaged. Try to learn when your hands and arms are relaxed. First of all, clench your fists, bend your elbows up, hold your arms together in front of your chest, and count to five. Then drop your arms to your side and unclench your fists, allowing your wrists to feel floppy and hands to rest with thumbs and fingers slightly apart and very slightly flexed.

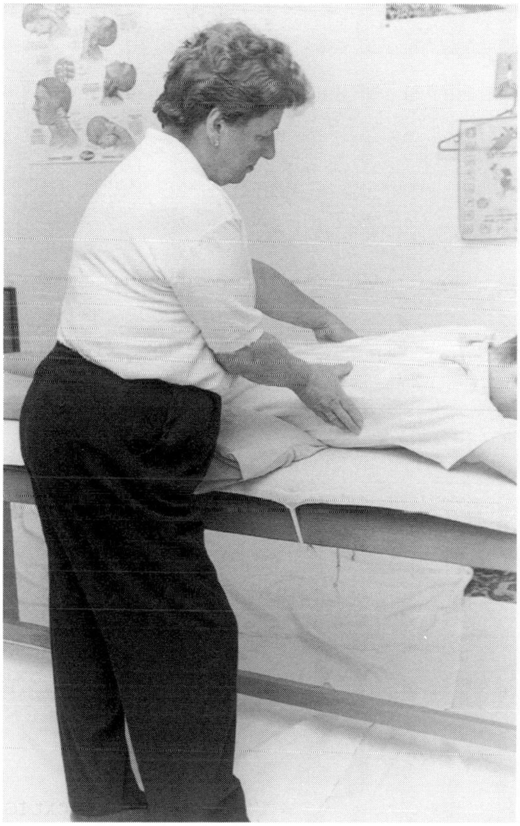

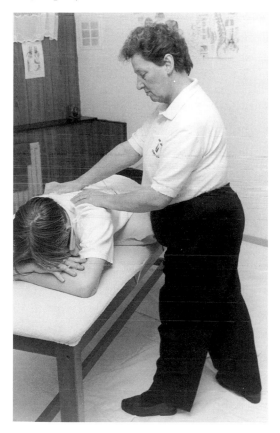

Fig 14. Optimum posture for massage – side view.

Fig 15. Optimum posture for massage – face on.

Palpation

Sense of touch has to become highly developed in the competent masseur. Only with practice can you increase your sense of touch and therefore your palpatory skills. It is essential to have a good basic knowledge of anatomical landmarks. Use your own body to familiarize your sense of touch. Feel the point of your elbow first with thumb tip, each finger pad in turn, then all fingers together and finally with the palm of your hand. Remember to do this with each hand in turn. Then repeat the exercise on your calf muscle, on your shin, on the front of your thigh, on the back of the thigh, on your abdomen and on your back, neck and face. Once you can begin to appreciate the differing textures and contours of the various body areas, start to palpate with your eyes closed and this will increase your skills even more. A good way to train sense of touch is the party game in which a bag is filled with various articles. Start with a tennis ball, an orange, a rubber ball, a cricket ball and a foam ball in the bag, close your eyes and pop your hand into the bag and try to identify which ball you are palpating. Then make the game more difficult by using smaller and smaller objects and using textures which are more closely related to each other.

As well as learning to increase your sense of touch you must also learn what is light contact and what constitutes heavy pressure. Not all participants will require or appreciate the same depth of massage, and what is light to one may appear heavy to another. Start by placing the pad of one thumb on the back of the opposite hand so that you can only just feel the contact, then gradually press in until the contact is actually unpleasant. Then grip your forearm between the thumb and first finger, initially so that you only just feel the contact and progressing to the unpleasant feel. When performing massage it can be equally unpleasant and unproductive to give too light pressure as to give too firm pressure. The first is sometimes referred to as 'skin polishing', which has no benefit at all and can be annoying, particularly to people who are ticklish. On the other hand, too firm pressure may well produce trauma and can be damaging. As a guideline it is good practice to ask the participant if your touch is at the correct depth for them and apply any alteration in tandem to their wishes. The only exception to this is if you feel that to go any deeper might cause actual tissue damage.

Only with practice will you appreciate the difference in depth of application, but learn to observe the reactions of the participant – a facial grimace, intake of breath or tensing of the tissue being treated indicates pain and therefore possibly too heavy massage or an area of pain indicative of an injury site. Wriggling and constant change of position is a sign of too light a touch.

PREPARATION OF THE PARTICIPANT

Always enquire if the participant has had massage before. Explain what you will be doing and be very specific as to what clothing needs to be removed and why.

In the Clinical Situation

1. For full body massage only pants or briefs should remain on and the participant should be given a full length towelling robe. This robe should be open at the front for frontal massage and changed to open at the back for back massage. **Remember that at all times the participant's modesty must be preserved**.
2. For full leg massage the upper body may be fully clad, but ensure that the participant is not going to become overwarm or chilled in the part not being massaged. Legs

should be completely exposed, trousers must be removed (not rolled up) and pants/briefs should be loose enough to allow access to lymph glands in the groin.

3. For lower leg massage trousers/track bottoms may be worn provided they can be loosely rolled above the knee without causing any restriction to circulation.

4. For foot massage the lower limb must be exposed, as in lower leg massage, so as to permit the strokes to reach the lymph glands behind the knee. During specific foot massage the lower leg must be covered with a blanket or towel.

5. For full arm massage the shoulder to the neck must be exposed with all shoulder straps removed.

6. For lower arm massage it is still necessary to remove clothing from the upper arm so as to enable strokes to reach the lymph glands under the armpit.

7. Hand massage should begin with general arm massage and end with the same, so removal of clothing is as above with the upper arm and forearm being covered with a blanket or towel during hand-specific massage.

8. Neck massage necessitates the removal of all clothing from the shoulder blades upwards. The participant's modesty is protected by specially made towelling robes which circle immediately below the armpits and fasten at the side. If these are not available a large bathsheet wrapped around and tucked in will suffice. It is important that the client feels this garment is secure as they will not relax if they feel it is going to slip.

9. Back massage requires all clothing except pants/briefs to be removed. It is necessary for pants/briefs to be able to be pushed down sufficiently to expose the gluteal cleft. The participant should be given a towelling gown to be worn back-to-front, thus exposing the back but adequately covering the front of the body.

10. Abdominal massage requires only the area from the lower ribs to the groin to be exposed. Pants/briefs and, for females, a bra that is not too tight or restrictive is worn and again a towelling robe.

At the Event – Track/Pitch Side

1. Full body massage will mean each area of the body being exposed as necessary and the rest being covered by towels/blankets or the participant's own clothing.

2. For full leg massage it is best to uncover only one limb at a time and keep track bottoms on the other limb until ready to massage it.

3. Lower leg massage is as above, treating one leg in turn and ensuring the other leg is well covered until being massaged.

4. Foot massage – again, one at a time and use clothing or towels/blankets to keep the rest of the body covered.

5. For full arm massage, slip off arm covering and push straps to one side, retaining clothing on the other arm.

6. For the lower arm, expose as above and cover the upper arm with a towel when not actually massaging it.

7. Hand massage – as above for full arm massage.

8. For neck massage, remove clothing and expose to shoulder blades and then redress tying track top/towel around under armpits.

9. For back massage, remove clothing to waist and redress with track top back to front, keep track bottoms on and push down, with towel tucked in as needed to treat lower back.

10. For abdominal massage leave track top and bottom on. Expose as needed, using towels tucked into waistband for protection.

It may not be possible at the venue to remove the person's clothing and massage may need to be applied with clothing still on. This does not give as good contact as on exposed skin, but may be the only option. In this instance ensure that the clothing does not create any friction to the part being massaged or give any danger of reaction to the masseur's hands. Light competition clothing, especially if made of lycra, is best, track suits are acceptable so long as they are not made of very shiny or thick material, but wet/waterproof clothing should be avoided.

PREPARATION OF THE MASSAGE VENUE/ENVIRONMENT

The environment to be used for sports massage will depend on two factors:

1. Whether the massage is to be administered in a clinical situation, such as in a specific sports medicine/massage clinic.
2. Whether the massage is to be administered at a sports arena or outdoor venue.

Massage in a Clinical Situation

It is most important that the room/area to be used for the application of massage is suitably prepared for this event. This is not difficult when one is working in a dedicated clinic area.

Preparation of a Room for Application of Sports Massage

The room temperature is vitally important. It must be comfortably warm so as to make the patient relax but not too hot for the masseur to work in, and there must be no draughts. Temperature should be easily controllable so that there is no risk of the client feeling cold or even cool during any of the massage.

It is important that the area is large enough to allow the masseur to move freely around all sides, top and bottom of the massage couch. As a massage couch measures 190–195cm (75–77in) long by 60–70cm (24–28in) wide, a good size for a massage cubicle is 290–300cm (115–120in) square. As well as a couch, the cubicle must contain a chair, wall hooks and hangers for the patient's clothing, clean towelling robes, shorts and towels, and a laundry basket so that each patient is reassured that the garments supplied to them are clean and removed for washing after use. The provision of a mirror and easy access to toilet facilities is essential, and the facility to shower both before and after massage can be very advantageous.

There should be a small trolley with the various massage coupling mediums, skin cleansers, cotton wool, tissues, extra towels and small pillows in the cubicle. If any aids to massage such as electrical applicators or wooden rollers are to be used these should be available and readily accessed. Electric power sockets should be at waist level to eliminate trailing cables.

Noise can negate the effects of relaxing massage. It is very much a matter of choice whether or not to have background music. Good practice is to enquire if the patient would wish to have music played and if possible to comply with their choice. But remember if their choice is unacceptable to the masseur the chance of a good massage is remote.

The client should be allowed to strip in privacy and put on a towelling gown, shorts or other modesty protector as appropriate. Cleanliness is obviously very important. If possible, a shower immediately prior to massage is excellent – only if the patient has showered immediately before massage and the masseur has asked them not to use any deodorants, talcum or perfumes can one be sure the skin is absolutely clean. After massage it is also helpful if the patient can shower if they so desire.

Treatment Couch

The best massage couch is one which can be raised and lowered either electrically or hydraulically. This ensures that the practitioner can have the height to suit all applications and also enable the patient to access the couch more readily if they have any physical problems (Fig 16). If a height-adjustable couch is not available it will be necessary to provide steps for the participant's use; also the practitioner may require some form of platform to give them the best working height (Fig 17).

Fig 16. Hydraulically operated massage couch.
Fig 17. *(Bottom)* Static couch with steps.

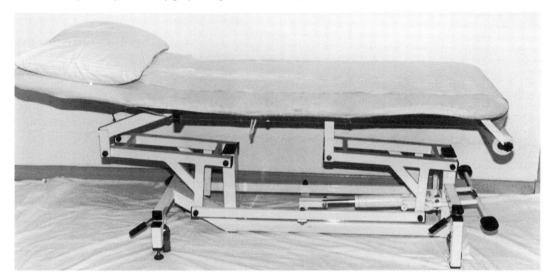

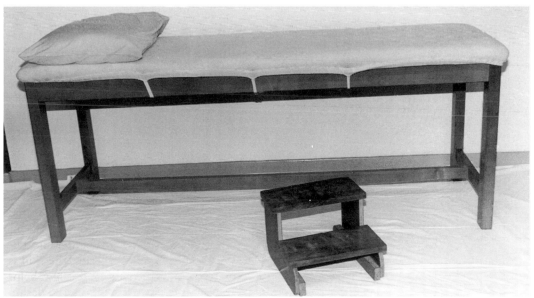

Soft Furnishings

- Terry couch covers.
- Paper couch rolls.
- Blankets.
- Towels – various sizes.
- Pillows – various shapes and sizes.
- Pillow cases.

Always allow adequate time at the end of the massage for the participant to ask any questions. Offer the shower facility and provide plenty of time for the patient to get dressed and prepare to depart without feeling rushed.

MASSAGE AT SPORTS ARENA OR OUTDOOR VENUE

The sports arena may be:

1. Indoors with facility provided.
2. Indoors with no facility provided.
3. Outdoors with facility provided.
4. Outdoors with no facility provided.

Indoors with Facility Provided

The indoor facility may well be a dedicated sports medicine clinic or sports massage facility. If so, all the criteria already described for the clinical situation would apply. This is the ideal situation if dealing with a club at their recognized training/competition venue. However, in the competition situation it is much more common to discover that a couch in the dressing room is all that is provided. At major events the provision of the massage facility will depend on the number of teams/people involved in the event and also the area/areas available. It may be that a sports hall will be designated as the massage venue. **This is a good area if there is screening providing individual treatment areas**

per team. Provision of a couch, chair and rubbish bin is about all one can hope for. It is also a bonus if there are hand-washing facilities in the vicinity, if not actually in the room provided. Many international sports bodies do have prepared lists of necessary provision for sports massage facilities at major events and a copy of these can be a help, but no guarantee that the items will be available.

Indoors with No Facility Provided

This tends to be the most common situation when travelling to sporting events. The first priority is to identify a suitable room/area to be used for the sports massage area. Look out for a changing room which can either double for some of the competitors to use or is close to where your team is going to be located. Remember if you are dealing with both sexes the facility must afford as much privacy as possible and preserve decency. The most difficult requirements are to observe both the participant's privacy and the basic rules of hygiene. Ambient temperature can also be a big problem – if the room is suitable but a bit cold accept the situation and be prepared for both participant and masseur to keep warm by using clothing, towels or whatever is available. It is possible to expose only small areas and use the participant's own clothing as previously described.

The first essential that the masseur must provide if intending to massage at sporting venues is a portable massage couch. There are many such couches on the market, but before you rush out and buy one, be sure you are aware of what you really require. The most important feature is portability. If the couch is too heavy for you to carry or too large for you to move without it trailing on the ground it is not suitable. A good portable couch, which must be steady enough when erected, will weigh in the region of 20kg (44lb). It

Fig 18. Portable couch.

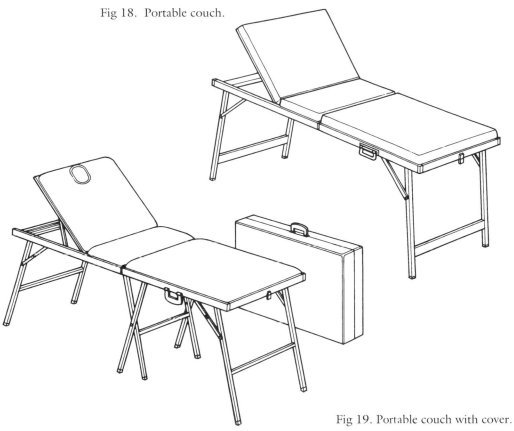

Fig 19. Portable couch with cover.

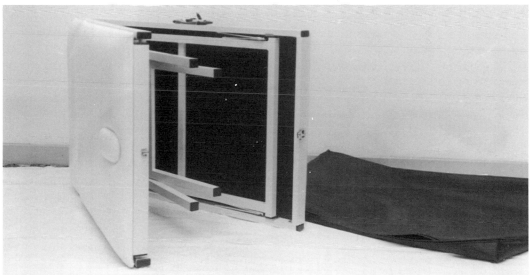

should have height adjustment, a facility to alter the backrest position and a breathing hole. Besides being stable when erected the couch should fold down easily. If you intend to travel by public transport, whether rail, coach or aeroplane, the couch needs to have a very good separate cover and be capable of withstanding abuse whilst being transported (Figs 18 & 19).

Inflatable pillows of varying sizes are useful and are the easiest to transport, but are not the most comfortable from the patient's point of view. A terry towelling plinth cover and a few towels will fit readily inside the portable couch.

All of your massage accoutrements, such as coupling media, tissues, cleansers and towels, need to be readily available in a large bag – remember you will have to be prepared to carry all this as well as the portable couch. (Tip – invest in a good set of luggage wheels and use these to transport all of your massage gear.)

If no portable couch is available, the masseur must utilize whatever 'prop' is to hand – changing room bench padded with blanket, towels or clothing, high-jump landing bed, spectators' seating, and so on. Only if there is absolutely nothing else to be found should the masseur and participant descend to the ground. The floor is very hard, of doubtful hygiene and massaging on your knees is not to be recommended. However, there may well be times when the masseur has to kneel on the ground – if so, be sure to use some item such as a pad to protect your knees and do not jeopardize your posture.

Outdoors with Facility Provided

At outdoor venues, especially when there are a large number of participating teams, the only facility may well be an overhead canvas area. Sometimes it may be a tented area with each team being allocated a tent for their exclusive use, or in really good situations it may be a Portakabin. If there is a Portakabin, the best will come equipped with water and therefore a hand-washing facility. Much more common is to find a tent or overhead canvas only. When faced with this situation try to choose the tent which gives the greatest protection from the sun and prevailing wind and is furthest away from any temporary toilet facility. Obviously a portable couch is essential and all the necessary towels and massage accoutrements described above. The possibility of hand-washing is likely to be very remote and it is essential that wet tissues are carried and used regularly to cleanse the hands and often the area to be massaged as well.

Outdoors with No Facility

This can try your ingenuity to the limit. If you have a portable couch, do try to set it up in an area where there is shade from the sun. At the start of the day it may seem quite pleasant to be outdoors in the fresh air with the sun shining down, but at the end of the afternoon after a full day in the sun you will be burnt to a frazzle as well as many of your participants being affected by the sun whilst receiving massage. **Remember some massage oils may encourage sunburn**. Again, only as a last resort should you attempt to administer massage with the competitor and masseur on the ground.

CHAPTER 2

Basic Rules of Sports Massage

Before embarking on the strokes and techniques used in sports massage the basic rules of such a regime must be addressed.

BASIC RULES OF SPORTS MASSAGE

1. Diagnosis.
2. History.
3. Assessment.
4. Contraindications.
5. Aims of treatment.
6. Position.
7. Materials.
8. Skin preparation.
9. Joint position.
10. Technique.
11. Check.
12. Clean up.
13. Warn participant.

Diagnosis

A dictionary definition of diagnosis is: *noun* 'the distinguishing of a disease by means of its symptoms'; *verb* 'to diagnose' 'to ascertain from symptoms as a disease'. My belief is that when giving sports massage, the issue of diagnosis will only apply if the massage is to be used to treat a sports injury, and the masseur doing this must be properly trained in anatomy, physiology, pathology and assessment. **It is vital that no masseur should ever attempt to diagnose without the proper training**. All masseurs should work within their own sphere of expertise. To provide adequate information on diagnosis this book would need to include a work the size of *Gray's Anatomy*. If a masseur is not trained to diagnose to a degree that would satisfy a court of law, their practice should not include diagnosis, and when injuries appear help should be sought from the appropriate professional. In many cases the masseur will treat the injury after it has been diagnosed by this professional and an excellent result will be obtained.

History

It is always good practice to obtain a full history – either relevant to a particular problem, or previous experience of and reaction to massage. A record card will be required to make notes and to store the information obtained (Figs 20 & 21).

Example Information Required on Record Card

- Participant's name, address, telephone number, sport, level of participation.
- Occupation.
- General practitioner's name, address, telephone number.
- Physiotherapist's name, address, telephone number.

MASSAGE RECORD   DATE:

NAME: DOB:
ADDRESS: TEL. NO:

OCCUPATION:
SPORT: PARTICIPATION LEVEL:

DOCTOR'S NAME: TEL. NO:
ADDRESS:

PHYSIOTHERAPIST'S NAME: TEL. NO:
ADDRESS:

COACH'S NAME: TEL. NO:
ADDRESS:

PREVIOUS INJURY:

PRESENT INJURY:

MASSAGE: HAD BEFORE? YES/NO
                                            ANY REACTION? YES/NO

IF REACTION WHAT:
KNOWN ALLERGIES:

                    ASSESSMENT

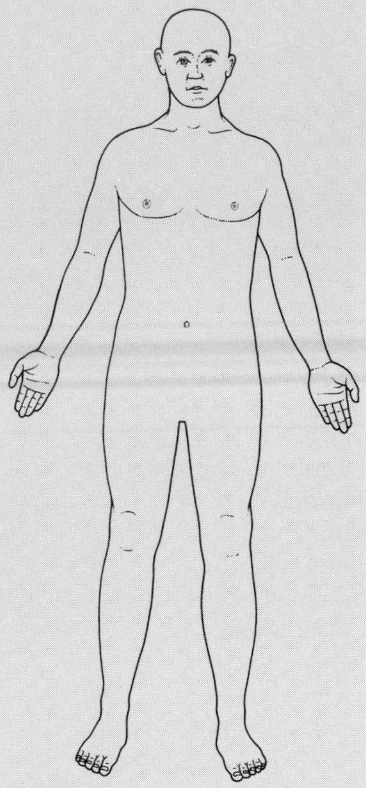

MASSAGE RECORD

DATE: MASSAGE USED: INITIALS:

Fig 20. *(Top)* Front of record card.   Fig 21. *(Above)* Back of record card.

MASSAGE RECORD

DATE: NAME: MASSAGE USED: INITIALS:

Fig 22. Sports venue record card.

- Coach's name, address, telephone number.
- Any current injury problem, treatment being given.
- Previous injury/injuries with dates if possible.
- Massage: previous massage – where, when, by whom, reaction to massage.
- Allergies.
- Relevant medical history – skin disorders, superficial infections, cuts, bruises, abrasions, unhealed scars, recent fractures, inflammation, especially acutely inflamed joints.
- Pregnancy, heavy menstruation, constipation.
- Cardio-vascular conditions, for example thrombosis, phlebitis, angina, hypertension.
- Any conditions being treated at the present time by a doctor, physiotherapist or other practitioner.
- Date of first contact.

At the sports venue it is not always possible to obtain or write down a complete history and on these occasions a shortened version (Fig 22) is used.

Assessment

Before embarking on any massage regime the masseur must have a good working knowledge of practical and surface anatomy and the relevant applied physiology. It is not possible to undertake a meaningful assessment if this knowledge is lacking. The first part of the masseur's assessment should be by observation:

- General observation of the participant's posture and movements on arrival for massage.
- Specific observation of a particular part of that area to be massaged.
- Questioning – adding to those already used in history taking, specific to the rea-

son for massage at that time. For example, where the client is in the training cycle, pre-, post- or inter-competition, and what stage of training – heavy, light, conditioning or resting.
- Movement – if giving general body massage – ascertain if any particular movements are giving a problem. For limb massage compare the participant's active movement of the limb in question with the opposite side – if there are any differences proceed to the passive range and compare again.
- Identification – bony points, tendons, ligaments and joint lines are all identified (Figs 23, 24 & 25). Any restrictions or limitations in joint movement (Fig 26) and the muscles (Figs 27 & 28) involved are identified.

If there is any problem in making an assessment and identification, help must be sought from the appropriate health professional.

Contraindications

It is important to remember that in some conditions massage may exacerbate problems and may even be dangerous – if in doubt, seek help.

Infections of the Skin

Bacterial infections of the skin. Boils and folliculitis (inflammation of the hair follicles) are the most common bacterial skin infections. Massage is not used because it can burst boils or blisters present in folliculitis. This leaves the skin open to further infections as well as producing pain. Impetigo is still a fairly common contagious infection found in athletes. Massage irritates the lesions and spreads the condition as well.

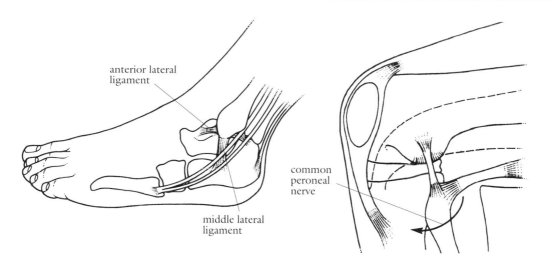

Fig 23. Surface anatomy left ankle lateral aspect.   Fig 24. Surface anatomy left knee lateral aspect.

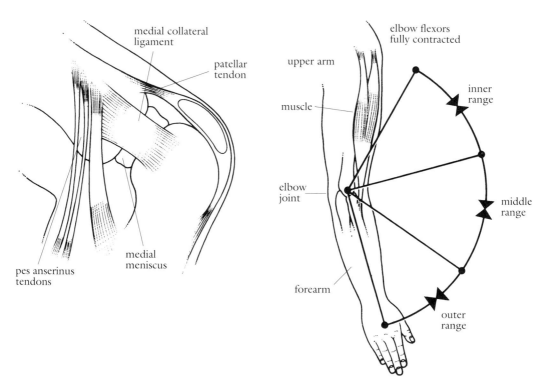

Fig 25. Surface anatomy left knee medial aspect.   Fig 26. Range of joint movement.

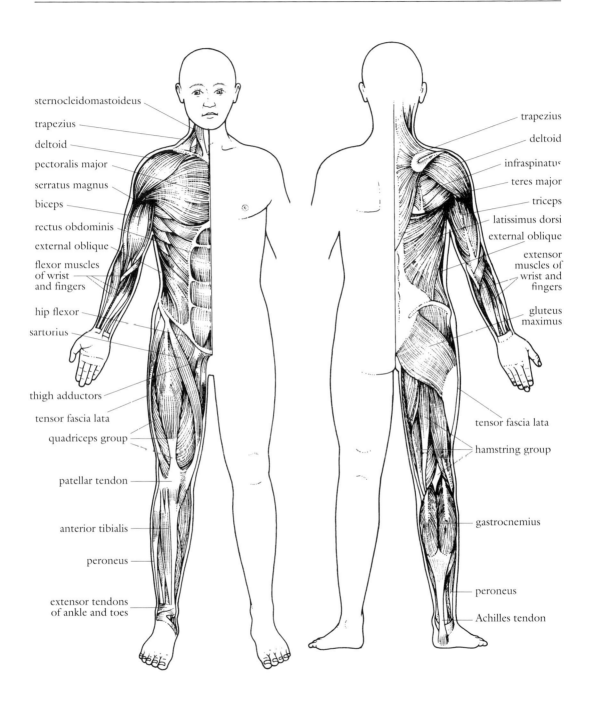

sternocleidomastoideus

trapezius

deltoid

pectoralis major

serratus magnus

biceps

rectus obdominis

external oblique

flexor muscles
of wrist
and fingers

hip flexor

sartorius

thigh adductors

tensor fascia lata

quadriceps group

patellar tendon

anterior tibialis

peroneus

extensor tendons
of ankle and toes

trapezius

deltoid

infraspinatus

teres major

triceps

latissimus dorsi

external oblique

extensor
muscles of
wrist and
fingers

gluteus
maximus

tensor fascia lata

hamstring group

gastrocnemius

peroneus

Achilles tendon

Fig 27. Muscular system – anterior view.   Fig 28. Muscular system – posterior view.

Fungal infections of the skin. Athlete's foot and ringworm are the most common fungal skin infections found in sports people. Massage tends to increase the irritation and there is a risk of transmission to the masseur.

Viral infections. Those most commonly found in sport are of the herpes (cold sore) family. These lesions are extremely tender and massage causes great irritation as well as risking transmission to the masseur. Warts and verrucae are also viral infections common in sport. Although massage does not directly affect these lesions unless they are bleeding, there is a great risk of the infection being transmitted to the masseur.

Open Wounds

Massage should not be used over any open wound, because of the risk of opening the wound more and the risk of transmission of infection. It is very common in many sports – for example, in track and field – to find many small spiking injuries. If these are open and weeping they should be avoided in any massage. **Care must be taken in selection of massage medium in these cases.**

Circulatory Problems

Bleeding disorders such as haemophilia, arteriosclerosis, artificial blood vessels, haemorrhage, thrombosis are all contraindications to massage. Massage increases blood flow and involves manipulation of blood vessels, both of which can adversely affect the above-mentioned circulatory problems. **If there is any history or doubt, seek proper medical help.**

Recent Injury

Any acute injury such as a muscle tear, tendon, ligament or connective tissue damage or bone injury, either fracture or periosteal damage, should not be massaged. Massaging too early in the healing process causes further damage to the fragile tissues that are involved in repair. This will not only delay the healing but can also restart bleeding and cause excess scar tissue to be formed. **As a rule of thumb, do not massage within 48 hours of known injury.** Then proceed with great care and very gentle strokes.

Tumours

Local massage produces mechanical stimulation which can speed up metabolism and so spread tumours.

Acute Inflammation

This condition can also be increased by massage.

Myositis Ossificans

This condition is not unusual in sports people. It occurs when bone is deposited within a muscle as a result of contusion and ensuing haematoma. The most common sites in sports participants are in the quadriceps and biceps muscles. Massage of these areas can produce further damage to the soft tissue surrounding the site of ossification and, if massage is particularly heavy and vigorous, it can separate small bony particles.

Diabetes

Although diabetes is not a complete contraindication to massage, care should be taken. It is not uncommon for the peripheral circulation to be affected in this condition, as a result of which skin and soft tissue are more easily damaged by massage.

Alteration of Skin Sensation

Loss of skin sensation, heightened sensation or presence of tingling, and pins and needles should all contraindicate massage. In certain instances massage may be given by the experienced practitioner, provided that the causes for the changes have been identified by the appropriate expert and no further contraindications are established.

Aims of Treatment

The aims of the massage will be dependent upon what type of sports massage is to be administered and at what stage of the training/competitive cycle this is taking place. Before the masseur can determine the aims of treatment he/she must be aware of the effects of massage.

It is now widely accepted and well-documented that massage does have therapeutic and reflex effects. According to Holey and Cook (1997): 'There are many postulated effects which are widely believed and documented throughout the massage literature. Unfortunately, not many of these have been substantiated scientifically.' The effects of the various massage strokes and techniques are dealt with later. The most important aims of sports massage are to:

- Help in the preparation for training or competition.
- Assist in the recovery from training or competition.
- Assist in the inter-competition preparations.
- Enhance a feeling of well-being.
- Specifically help in the stretching programme.
- Specifically treat an injury, but only after this has been accurately diagnosed and sanctioned by the appropriate medical person.

It is vital to ascertain from the participant what type of massage they require at any particular time and then draw up the aims of treatment accordingly.

Position

As previously stated in the preparation chapter, it cannot always be guaranteed that there will be a massage couch available. When using massage in sport *always* ensure that the masseur is positioned in such a manner as to be able to perform all necessary techniques with the greatest ease. Great care must be taken to keep the recipient warm and comfortable with decency maintained. The masseur has the responsibility to protect their own back by maintaining a good and safe working posture. It may be necessary to kneel on the ground, but as previously noted this really is only as a last resort.

Materials (Lubricants)

The chapter on preparation has already dealt with the couches, pillows, covers, towels and so on that are necessary to perform massage. The other materials used are the lubricants. There are many and varied types of massage oils, creams and powders available and the use of essential oils in aromatherapy is growing daily. The first simple advice is to ensure that the lubricant selected is acceptable to both masseur and recipient and meets the requirements of the aims of massage.

It is absolutely essential that the masseur is aware of all the ingredients contained in any lubricant they may use. Remember that some massage oils contain nut oils and so may be catastrophic if applied to a person with an allergy to nuts. Very hairy skin will tend to be irritated by the use of powder or insufficient oils during massaging. Masseurs who suffer from sweaty hands may find that oils increase this tendency and a light powder is preferable.

The ambient temperature and weather conditions may affect the choice of lubricant. Very cold weather may make some creams too solid to apply easily, while too much heat will have the opposite effect and often turn oils and creams into runny liquids. Powders used on sweaty skins will help to dry them, but can also form lumps and drag on hair and skin with the resultant risk of folliculitis.

Ice massage will be dealt with later, but is a useful medium in certain circumstances. Water alone or soapy water can be very good lubrication especially if dealing with very hot or dry scaly skin. In the latter instance the addition of oil to the soapy water is extremely beneficial.

Included in materials/lubricants must be cleaning agents. It is most important that a sports competitor does not enter the arena dripping with oil or any other massage lubricant. Where possible, a shower immediately after the massage is best, but obviously at the venue, during training and/or competition this may well be impracticable and undesirable. Moist tissues and assorted small pieces of towelling are very useful. These can be used to wipe down the areas massaged either on their own or in conjunction with a mild astringent. (Tip – make up your own from a mixture of rose water and cleansing lotion.)

Skin Preparation

When performing any massage, the skin area to be treated should be examined:

1. *Ask.* Find out by questioning if the participant has any tender areas, any injury they are aware of, or any other relevant information, for example, old scars, varicose veins, reactions of any kind to lubricants.
2. *Look.* Observe the condition of the skin. Is it dry, oily, hairy (may recently have been shaved), wet (with water and/or sweat), sand-covered (very common in long and triple jumpers)? Are there any bruises, cuts, shaving nicks, spike injuries, lumps of known or unknown origin, spots or rashes present? Also check for any swelling, tension or redness and remember if the training or competition has been outdoors sunburn may be starting or be present.
3. *Palpate (Feel).* Run your hand over the areas to be massaged and assess the temperature and note if there is any reaction from the recipient. Find out if this reaction is caused by pain or if the area may just be ticklish.

All areas of skin should be as clean as possible and any extraneous matter removed prior to application of the massage. Where there are open wounds, spike injuries and/or razor nicks these should be protected with appropriate dressings and care taken not to infiltrate that area with any massage lubricant.

Joint Position

Sports massage will not produce the best effect if the participant is not fully supported and in as relaxed position as possible for the technique to be administered.

Whole Leg Massage

Front (anterior) aspect of the leg. The participant is as flat as is comfortable on their back (supine). Do not raise the back of the couch more than 40 to 45 degrees as this will impede drainage from the limb to the glands in the groin. If elevation of the limb is required use a pillow/pillows or where possible raise the lower end of the couch (Fig 29).

Back (posterior) aspect of the leg. The participant is flat on their front (prone). Put the pillow under both ankles to allow flexion at the knees (Fig 30). If agreeable to both masseur and participant the masseur may perch on the

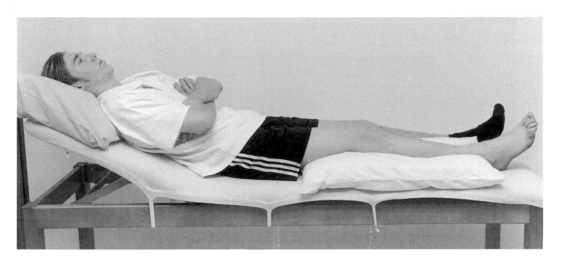

Fig 29. Using pillow to elevate lower limb.

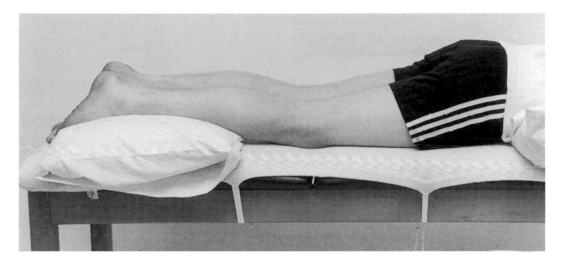

Fig 30. Prone lying with pillow supporting lower limbs.

couch and rest the ankle on the masseur's shoulder (this is very useful at venues with no pillows available) (Fig 31).

Below Knee/Above Knee Massages

The positions are as above with only the area to be massaged being exposed.

Whole Arm Massage

If done sitting, the arm should be supported on a pillow resting on a small arm table, so that both anterior and posterior aspects can be reached (Fig 32).

If done lying, the participant is prone or supine depending on the surface to be treated.

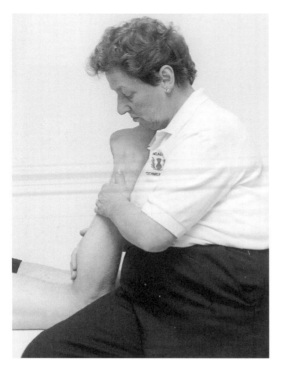

Fig 31. Use of masseur's shoulder to support lower limb.

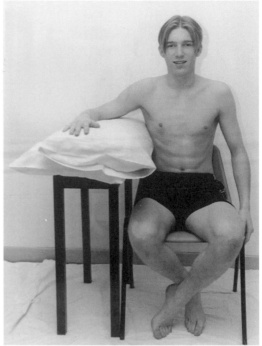

Fig 32. Sitting with arm supported.

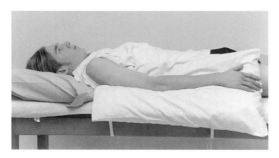

Fig 33. Lying arm supported for arm massage.

The arm is supported on a pillow alongside the trunk (Fig 33).

Forearm Massage

This is generally done with the participant sitting and supported as described above.

Upper Back Massage, Thoracic Area and Buttocks

The participant is prone with a pillow under the abdomen and another pillow under both lower legs. Use the breathing hole in the couch if applicable, or if not, a small pillow to support the forehead (Fig 34).

Neck, Cervical Area/Posterior Shoulder Girdle

The participant is prone lying as above. For some treatments, the participant should be supine with only a small pillow under the knees. If sitting, he/she should be on a stool or massage chair with head resting in forearms on a pillow (it is important that the back is straight and neck not flexed) (Fig 35).

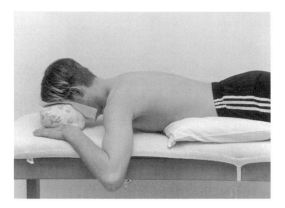

Fig 34. Position for upper back massage.

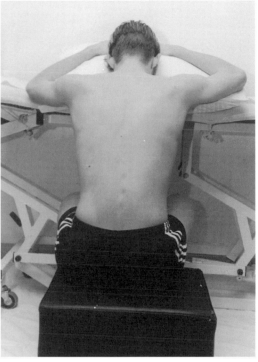

Abdominal Massage

The recipient should be supine with small pillows under the head and knees.

Hand Massage

The participant should be in a sitting position, hands resting on a pillow supported on the table, their knees, or the masseur's knees.

Fig 35. Sitting, back straight, neck not flexed position for neck massage.

Foot Massage

The recipient should be in a sitting position, on a chair with the leg and foot supported on a footstool and pillow, or in a sitting position on a couch with a pillow under the leg to be treated.

Obviously, at track side, pitch side or venue the necessary treatment couch, chair or other supports may not be available. In these instances the masseur must be adaptable and use whatever may be available. **However, always ensure that the recipient is comfortable and the joints are supported in as comfortable and stress-free position as can be attained**.

Technique

The most commonly used techniques in sports massage have their origins in Swedish massage. A list of these techniques follows. Details of each stroke, application and effects are dealt with in later chapters. These are:

Stroking Manipulations

(a) Effleurage.
(b) Stroking.

Pressure Manipulations or Petrissage

(a) Kneading.
(b) Picking up.

(c) Wringing.
(d) Rolling.

Frictions

(a) Circular.
(b) Transverse.

Tapotement

(a) Hacking.
(b) Clapping.
(c) Beating.
(d) Pounding.

Shaking

(a) Shaking.
(b) Vibration.

Other Techniques Used in Sports Massage

(a) Acupressure.
(b) Trigger pointing.

Check

Most sports people are extremely knowledgeable about their own body and preparation for activity. However, it is always good practice to check that you are in fact administering the type of massage required. Ask the participant if the massage is deep enough, too deep or not deep enough. Be ready to alter the depth to satisfy their requirements. **However, never change the depth of a massage if you feel this will be contraindicated**. If the participant requests a deeper massage and you feel there is any contraindication, such as a recent injury, or activity is very close, then be prepared to explain your reasons. If the person still insists refer on to a medical practitioner. Always check how much time the person has before they need to warm up, report or whatever is next on their agenda.

Clean Up

Participants cannot enter the competition or training area covered in oil, cream or powder. Oily legs or arms can transfer oils to hands with disastrous results if the participant needs to catch a ball or tackle an opponent. If the massage has been administered indoors in the clinic or a specific massage room, there should be shower facilities as previously described. At the pitch/track side, wet wipes, astringent lotion and towels will be required to ensure the skin is as free from lubricant as possible.

Warn Participant

Even if the participant has frequent massages, be sure to remind them what to expect as a result of each massage session: for example, pre-competition a massage is stimulating but cannot replace the proper warm-up and preparation prior to activity, whereas post-competition it does not replace cool-down and certain strokes may leave tenderness.

Whatever massage programme is being administered, you should always be confident that you know why you are performing that particular regime. You must have an accurate diagnosis available, proper history recorded, have checked all contraindications and discussed the aims of the treatment with the participant. The position for both masseur and participant must be the best possible and safest obtainable in the situation where the massage is to be performed. Materials must be appropriate, skin preparation before and after massage must be carried out. Joint position and techniques must not be compromised in even the most difficult of venues. Always check that the participant is contented with the procedure and is well aware of what to expect after the massage. **If in doubt seek the correct medical advice from a medical practitioner or chartered physiotherapist**.

CHAPTER 3

Sports Massage Techniques

Massage techniques most frequently used in sport can be listed under six headings.

SPORTS MASSAGE TECHNIQUES

1. Stroking Manipulations.
2. Pressure Manipulations or Petrissage.
3. Frictions.
4. Tapotement.
5. Shaking.
6. Acupressure and Trigger Pointing.

Stroking Manipulations

There are two categories of manipulation under this heading: effleurage and stroking.

Effleurage

Description of manipulation: This is a stroking movement usually performed from distal to proximal part of the body, ending in the appropriate lymph drainage area. It may be centripetal (towards the heart) (Fig 36), uni-

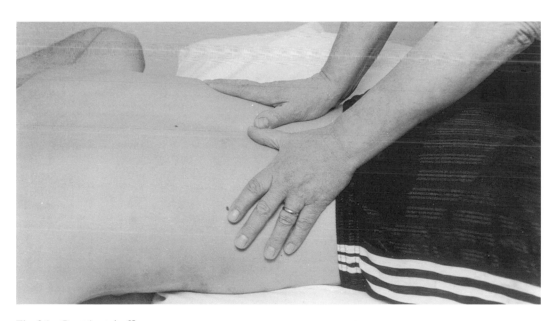

Fig 36. Centripetal effleurage.

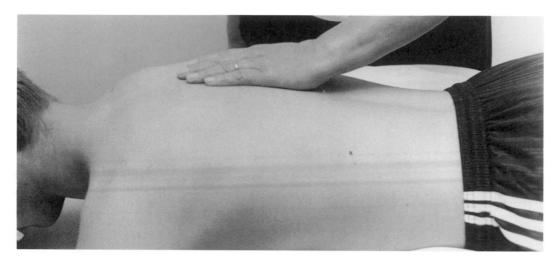

Fig 37. Unidirectional effleurage.

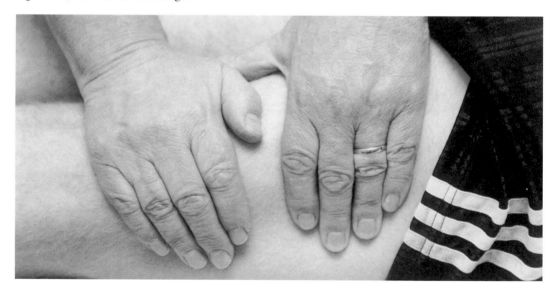

Fig 38. Multidirectional effleurage.

directional (Fig 37), multidirectional (Fig 38), circular (Fig 39), figure seven (Fig 40), figure eight (Fig 41) or T-shaped (Fig 42).

Depth: The depth needs to be sufficient to influence the onward flow of the superficial vessels, grade 1; affecting deeper vessels, grade 2; reinforced, grade 3.

Performance: This can be single whole hand (Fig 43), double whole hand (Fig 44), reinforced two hands (Fig 45), or one, two or

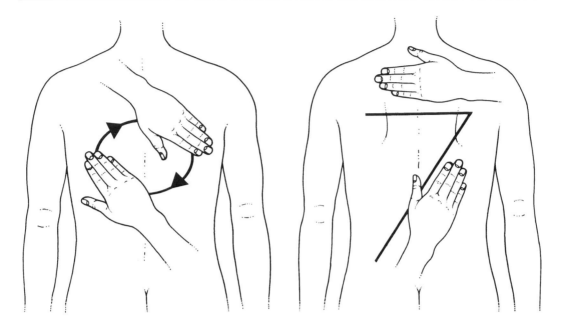

Fig 39. Circular effleurage.

Fig 40. Figure seven effleurage.

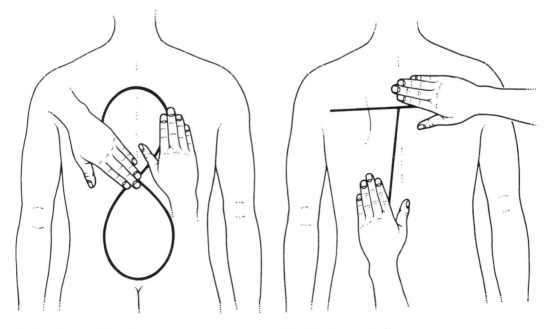

Fig 41. Figure eight effleurage.

Fig 42. T-shaped effleurage.

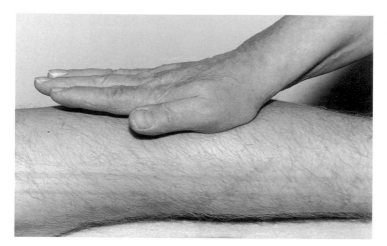

Fig 43. Single whole-hand effleurage.

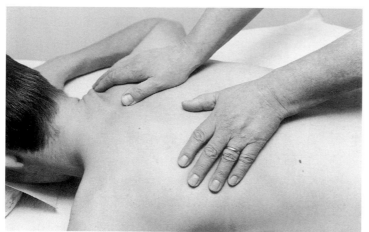

Fig 44. Double whole-hand effleurage.

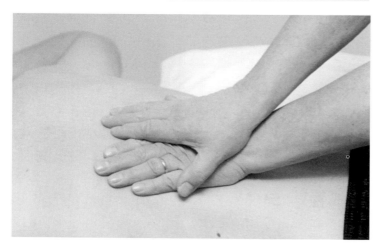

Fig 45. Reinforced two-handed effleurage.

three fingers or the thumb (Figs 46, 47, & 48).

Usage: At the start of massage, in between other manipulations, at the end of massage.

Effects:

- Superficial blood flow is hastened – grade 1.
- Lymph drainage is accelerated – all grades.
- Deep blood flow is increased – grade 2 and reinforced.

- Vasodilatation occurs in massage area – all grades.
- Sedative/decrease in muscle tone – grade 1.
- Stimulatory/increase in muscle tone – grade 2 and reinforced.
- Mobility of soft superficial tissues is increased – grade 1.
- Mobility of deeper tissues increased – grade 2 and reinforced.

Precautions: Be sure to apply adequate lubricant to allow smooth movement over skin at all depths.

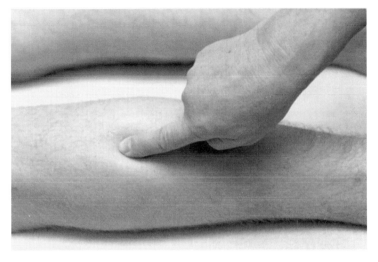

Fig 46. One finger effleurage.

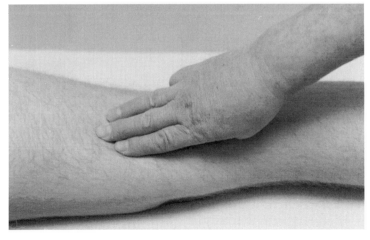

Fig 47. Three finger effleurage.

Stroking

Description of manipulation: The main difference between effleurage and stroking is the depth and direction. Traditional Swedish massage describes stroking as being performed from proximal to distal. In sports massage stroking may be centripetal (as Fig 36), centrifugal (away from the heart) (Fig 49), and cross-over.

Depth: Grade 1 contact is so very light as to give a sedative effect. Grade 2 is slightly firmer so as to produce minimal effect on superficial vessels.

Performance: This can be whole hand (as Fig 43), whole hand right then left (Fig 50), pad of finger, thumb, one, two or alternate (Fig 51), or thousand hands (Fig 52). In the thousand hands manipulation, one hand is used to perform a short stroke, the second hand then performs the same movement overlapping the first.

Grade 2 stroking can be whole hand one or two (Fig 53), whole hand right then left (Fig 54), pad of finger or thumb (as Fig 51), ulnar-

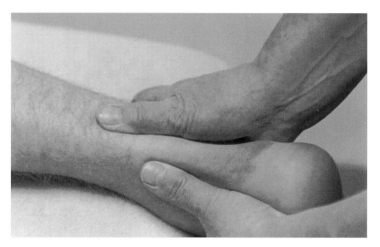

Fig 48. Thumb effleurage.

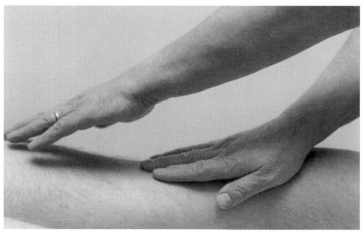

Fig 49. Stroking – centrifugal – both hands moving down leg.

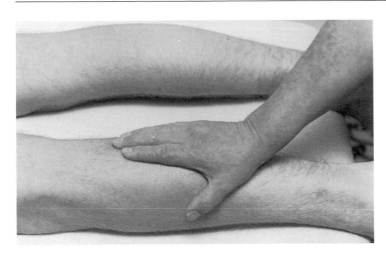

Fig 50. Whole right-hand stroking.

Fig 51. Finger and thumb stroking.

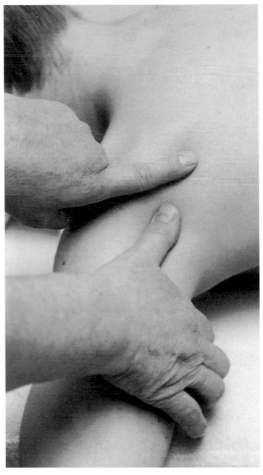

surface of fist (Fig 55), ulnar border of palm (Fig 56), heel of palm (Fig 57), ulnar border of forearm (Fig 58) or elbow (Fig 59).

Usage: To accustom participant to touch, to apply massage lubricant or at end of massage session.

Effects: The effects of Grade 1 are sedative, decreasing muscle tone, especially if performed slowly. Grade 2 hastens superficial blood flow and accelerates lymph drainage. It is stimulative, especially if performed briskly.

Precautions: The usual contraindications apply. It is also very easy to feel ticklish if insufficient pressure and contact are applied.

Pressure Manipulations or Petrissage

There are four categories under the heading of petrissage: kneading; picking up; wringing; and rolling.

In all four petrissage manipulations the soft tissues, that is, superficial tissue, muscle tissue and ligaments, are compressed and lifted. They may also be squeezed and rolled against themselves or underlying structures.

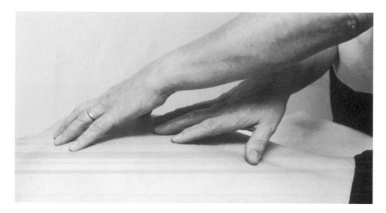

Fig 52. Thousand hand stroking.

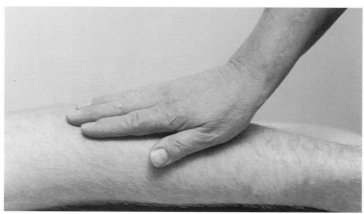

Fig 53. Grade 2 whole-hand stroking.

Kneading

Description of manipulation: The tissues are compressed against the underlying structure in this manipulation. The action for kneading is a circular movement and may be performed proximal to distal or distal to proximal.

Depth: Grade 1 is sufficient to influence superficial vessels and compress superficial soft tissues on underlying structures. Grade 2 is sufficient to affect deeper tissue drainage and compress deep tissue structures on underlying structures. Grade 3 is reinforced or superimposed as much as can be tolerated by the participant. It also affects deep structures and may cause compression onto bony structures.

Performance: The palmar aspect of the whole hand is employed, one or two hands, or alternate (Figs 60 & 61). A circle is performed by the hand with pressure on the upward part of the circle for about one quarter of the circumference (Fig 62). The hand must remain in full contact for the remainder of the circle and only be lifted to move on to perform the next circle.

- Palm only – either one hand, both or alternate (Figs 63 & 64) – very good on limbs.
- Finger kneading – using all of the fingers or combinations of one, two, three or four fingers (Fig 65).
- Finger pad or thumb pad kneading (Fig 66).

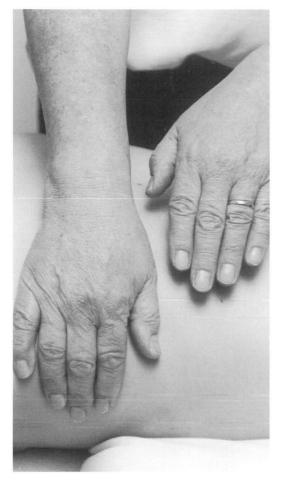

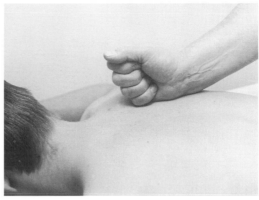

Fig 55. Grade 2 ulnar surface of the fist stroking.

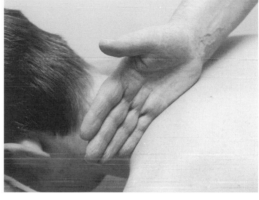

Fig 56. Grade 2 ulnar border of the palm stroking.

Fig 54. Grade 2 whole-hand right then left stroking.

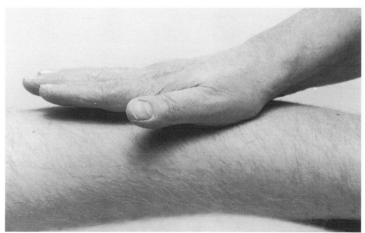

Fig 57. Grade 2 heel of palm stroking.

41

Fig 58. Grade 2 ulnar border of forearm stroking.

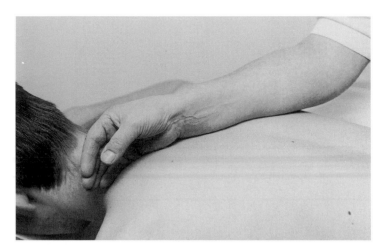

Fig 59. Grade 2 elbow stroking.

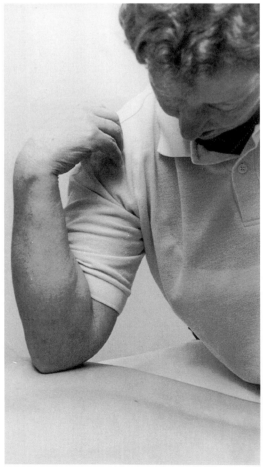

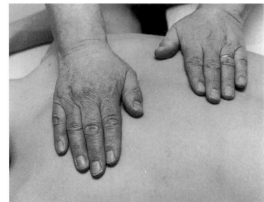

Fig 60. Palmar aspect two-handed kneading.

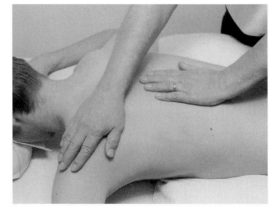

Fig 61. Alternate hand kneading.

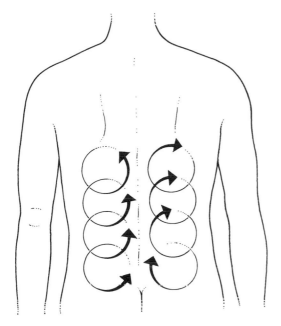

Fig 62. Direction of pressure in kneading.

Fig 63. Single-hand palm kneading.

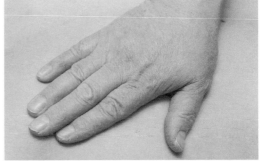

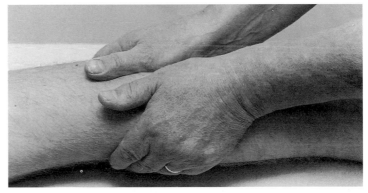

Fig 64. Double-hand palm kneading.

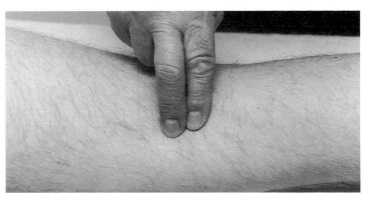

Fig 65. Finger kneading.

- Finger tip or thumb tip kneading (Fig 67).
- Reinforced or superimposed kneading – may be performed in any of the above manipulations (Fig 68).

Usage: This is used as part of sports massage to help mobilize soft tissues especially after other manipulations have accustomed the area to touch and induced relaxation in the tissues.

Effects

- Stimulates venous and lymphatic flow at all grades.
- Increases mobility of fibrous tissues at all grades.
- Helps interchange of tissue fluids at all grades.
- Helps prepare soft tissues for stretching and warm-up procedures at all grades.

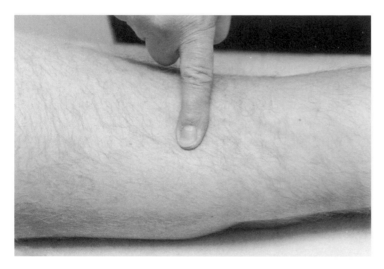

Fig 66. Finger pad kneading.

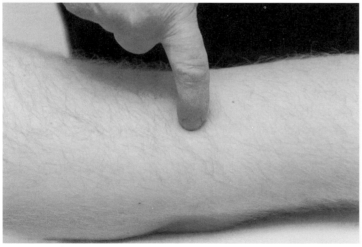

Fig 67. Fingertip kneading.

- Helps the removal of waste products at all grades.
- Increases strength and length of connective tissues at all grades.

Precautions: The usual contraindications apply. Be very careful not to compress too heavily, especially if the participant has just trained or competed or is about to do so. Also take care not to nip tissue by squeezing too hard.

Picking Up

Description of manipulation: The tissues are again compressed against underlying structures, then 'picked up' – lifted, squeezed and released. The movement is performed down a limb from proximal to distal; neck and shoulders are from occiput to axilla; on the back from cervical to lumbar region; and across the buttocks from central spine to lateral.

Depth: Grade 1 is sufficient to influence superficial vessels and compress superficial soft tissues on underlying structures. Grade 2 is sufficient to affect deeper tissue drainage and compress deep tissue structures on underlying structures. Grade 3 is only applicable to dou-ble-handed manipulation, as it will only be tolerated on very muscular areas. Do not perform more than can be tolerated by the participant as it affects deep structures and can cause compression onto bony structures.

Performance: Single-hand C-shape (Fig 69), double-hand alternate C-shape (Fig 70), single-hand V-shape (Fig 71), double-hand V-shape (Fig 72). For the C-shape, the hand is held with the thumb away from the palm to make the web between it and the first finger form a C-shape (as Fig 70). For the V-shape, the thumb is adjusted to make the web form a V-shape (as Fig 71). The elbows should be bent slightly and held away from the body at a comfortable position. The web of the hand forming the C or V must maintain contact with the participant's skin throughout the whole manipulation. The wrists should be held extended. Picking up takes place by performing a compressing and then lifting action. Full grade 3 depth is achieved by using transfer of body weight from the back to the front leg (Fig 73).

Usage: Picking up aims to assist mobilization of soft tissues, and is especially effective when used after effleurage and kneading.

Fig 68. Reinforced kneading.

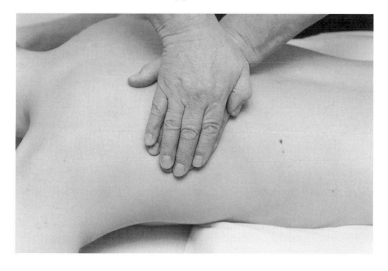

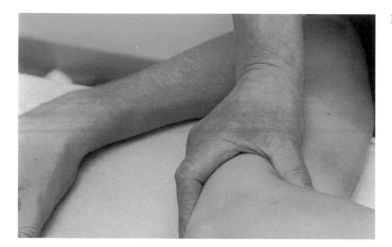

Fig 69. Picking up, C-shape.

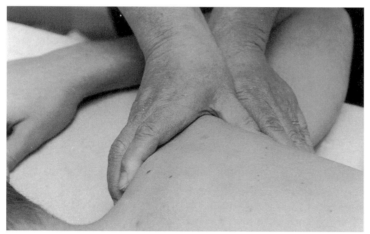

Fig 70. Picking up, double-handed C-shape.

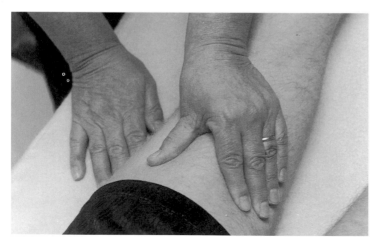

Fig 71. Picking up, V-shape.

Fig 72. Picking up, double-handed V-shape.

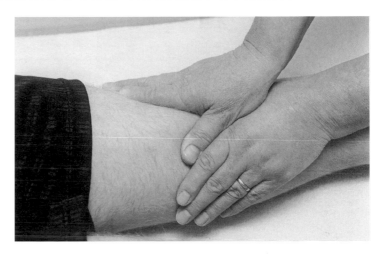

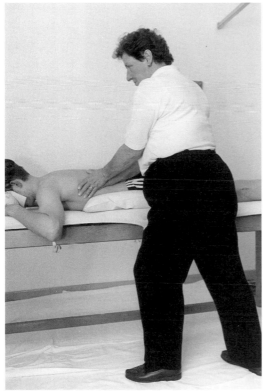

Fig 73. Transfer of body weight from back to front leg.

Effects: As stated for kneading above.

Precautions: Usual contraindications apply. Be very sure there is absolutely no risk of any soft tissue trauma if used inter- or post-competition or training. Note that if skin contact is lost during performance of manipulation a pinching action will result.

Wringing

Description of manipulation: The tissues are compressed against underlying structures, then one hand pulls towards the masseur and the other hand pushes away.

Depth: Grade 1 is as in kneading and picking up. It is usual to use fingers and thumbs only unless wishing to manipulate skin wringing on a larger area (such as back or shoulder girdle) when full hands are used. For grade 2, as in kneading and picking up, use the whole hand. Note that there is no grade 3, as it would be too painful for the participant to tolerate.

Performance: For finger/thumb wringing (Fig 74), the fingers and thumb are used to compress the tissues between them, then this

47

tissue is lifted and pulled towards you with one hand and pushed away from you with the other. For grade 1 hand wringing see Fig 75; for grade 2 hand wringing see Fig 76.

Usage: Wringing is used as part of sports massage to assist mobilization of tissues, and is best performed towards the end of a sequence prior to final effleurage.

Effects: As stated for kneading. It can help separate superficial and deep adherent tissues.

Precautions: Usual contraindications apply. Be aware of the risk of any tissue damage or injury post-event/training. Do not grasp tissue too tightly as this produces a nipping effect.

Rolling

Description of manipulation: Both hands are used for rolling. Contact is made with both palms, the thumbs are held away from the fingers, and the tips of the thumbs touch each other with a small space between the

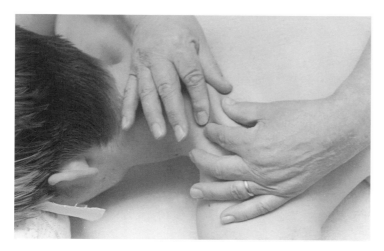

Fig 74. Finger/thumb wringing.

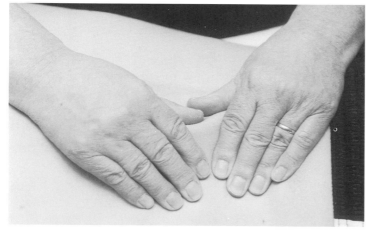

Fig 75. Grade 1 hand wringing.

fingertips (Fig 77). The fingers pull the tissue towards the thumbs (Fig 78) and then the thumbs squeeze and lift to push the tissue away (Fig 79). In the muscle rolling manipulation the roll of tissue is not so obvious and the action is more push with the thumbs and pull back with the fingers (Figs 80 & 81).

Depth: For grade 1, skin rolling only, which involves lifting only very superficial tissues. For grade 2, muscle rolling, which involves lifting muscle tissue and affecting deeper structures. Note that there is no grade 3, as it would be too painful.

Performance: skin rolling is shown in Figs 77, 78 and 79. It is important to stand facing the area being manipulated. Keep the palms in contact, pull the skin towards you, then push towards the fingers with squeeze and lift. Expect mobile skin to lift and roll over your fingers. Your palm lifts to accommodate the movement (Figs 82 & 83).

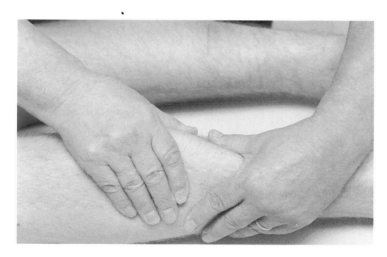

Fig 76. Grade 2 hand wringing.

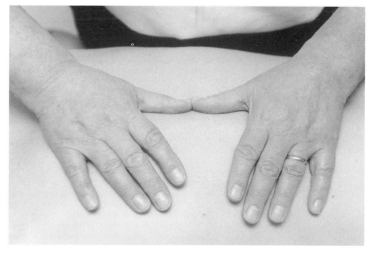

Fig 77. Skin rolling – tips of thumbs touching.

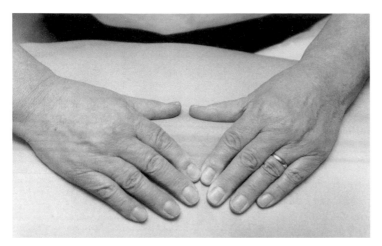

Fig 78. Skin rolling – fingers pull tissue towards thumbs.

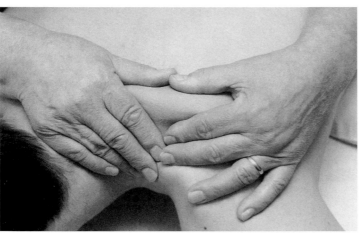

Fig 79. Skin rolling – thumbs squeeze and lift to push tissue away.

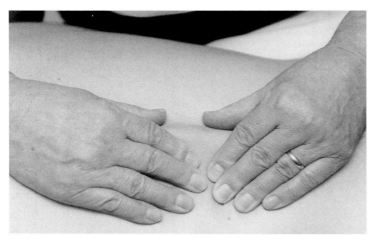

Fig 80. Muscle rolling – push with thumbs.

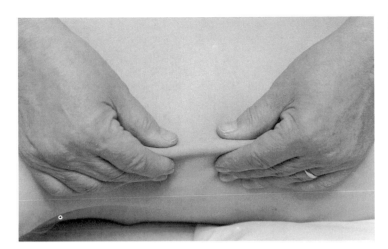

Fig 81. Muscle rolling – pull back with fingers.

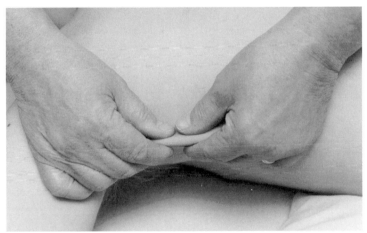

Fig 82. Muscle rolling – mobile skin lift palm.

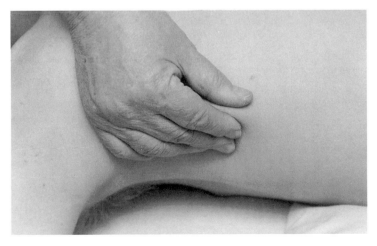

Fig 83. Muscle rolling – lifting action.

Muscle rolling is shown in Figs 80 and 81. Again, it is important to stand facing the area and to transfer body weight forwards and backwards with the direction of the manipulations.

Usage: The purpose of rolling is to assist mobilization of soft tissues. It is best performed after effleurage and then immediately stroked or effleuraged at the end of the rolling technique.

Effects: These are as stated for kneading plus it mobilizes scar tissue and, when performed slowly, has a stretch effect on the tissues being manipulated.

Precautions: The usual contraindications apply. Care must be taken not to be too violent or to nip the tissues when working on recent scarring.

Frictions

There are two main categories under this manipulation, circular friction and transverse friction.

Circular Friction

Description of manipulation: Pressure is applied to the area to be treated, and a small, circular manipulation is performed at a gradually increasing depth for two to five rotations. Then pressure is released and manipulation repeated on the same spot or adjacent tissue.

Depth: There is no grade 1, as this is a manipulation to affect deeper tissues. Grade 2 pressure is sufficient to affect deep tissues and cause compression. At grade 3 it is reinforced to affect deeper structures and may compress to bony tissues.

Performance: Fingertips are used. Only fingertip or tips are to cover the area; the rest of the hand must not touch the skin. Compression is applied and small, circular movements are performed at increasing depth, from once to five times (Fig 84).

When using thumb tip/tips, the area is covered only by thumb tip or tips. Again, the tissue is compressed and a circular action performed at increasing depth for two to five rotations (Fig 85).

When using reinforced circular friction, either the fingertip or thumb tip is covered by the adjoining digit or by those of the other hand and a circular action is repeated as above (Fig 86).

Usage: Circular friction is used as part of sports massage to restore tissue mobility and remove waste products. It is best used post competition and training.

Effects: It stimulates circulation locally, restores tissue mobility, and helps remove waste products.

Precautions: The usual contraindications apply. Do not use any lubricant as the manipulation does not require any finger movement across the skin. Never use if you suspect the possibility of recent soft tissue damage.

Transverse Frictions

Description of manipulation: This manipulation is frequently called 'Cyriax frictions', as Dr Cyriax first described the manipulation. The fingertip/tips or thumb tip/tips are used and may be reinforced. The finger/s or thumb/s is/are placed on the tissue, at 90 degrees to the tissue and pressure is applied, then a forwards and backwards motion is performed across the structure. **It is important that the participant must be advised that this will produce pain.**

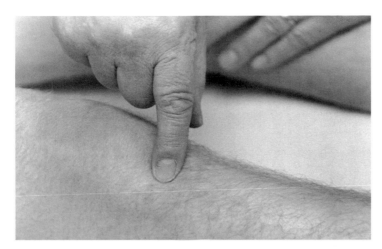

Fig 84. Circular fingertip friction.

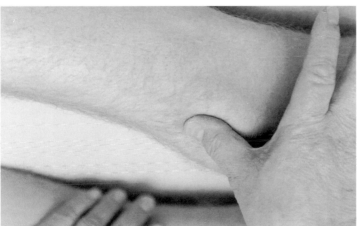

Fig 85. Circular thumb tip friction.

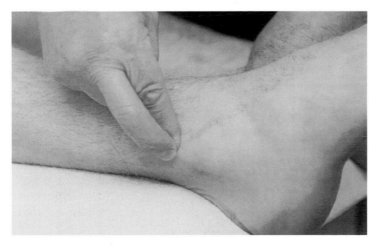

Fig 86. Circular reinforced fingertip friction.

Depth: This is performed to grade 3 only, and must be as deep as can be tolerated/achieved.

Performance: Finger or thumb tip is applied at 90 degrees to the tissue and pressure applied, a forwards and backwards action is performed with increasing depth, to the maximum that can be tolerated by the participant. This must be maintained for at least two minutes (Fig 87). The finger or thumb tip can be reinforced with another digit and the action performed as above (Fig 88).

Usage: This technique is used as a specific treatment for tendon, ligament, musculotendinous junctions and muscle tissue.

Precautions: The usual contraindications apply. The participant must be warned that the manipulation will produce pain until numbing is achieved. Transverse friction should be used only when accurate diagnosis has been given by a properly qualified practitioner, whether medical or a physiotherapist. Note that the skin must move with the finger/thumb tip or bruising and blistering may occur.

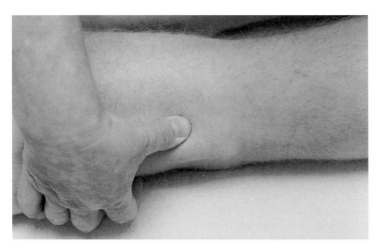

Fig 87. Transverse friction.

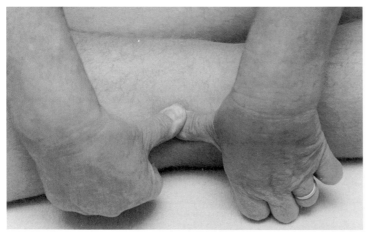

Fig 88. Transverse reinforced friction.

Tapotement

There are four main categories of manipulation under this heading which are used in sports massage: hacking; clapping; beating; and pounding.

Hacking

Description of manipulation: In this manipulation the area to be treated is hit by the medial border of the hands or fingers.

Depth: Grade 1 uses only medial borders of fingers; grade 2 uses medial borders of hands and fingers; grade 3 uses medial borders of hands and fingers slowly and deeply to produce mechanical effects on hollow organs (such as the lungs) – this is not really applicable to sports massage.

Performance: The masseur must stand with his or her shoulders over the area to be treated. Arms are abducted (away from body), elbows bent to almost 90 degrees (Fig 89) and wrists are extended with fingers relaxed (Fig 90). In grade 1 hacking (Fig 90), the fingers of one hand and then the other alternately make

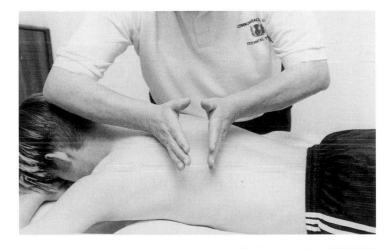

Fig 89. Elbow position for hacking.

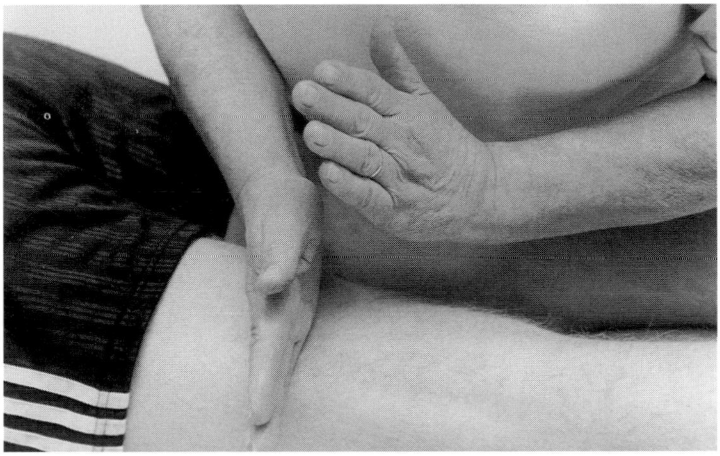

Fig 90. Grade 1 hacking, using fingers.

contact lightly and quickly (*see* practice on a pillow, Fig 9).

In grade 2 hacking, the stance, arm and wrist position are as grade 1, but the outer border of the hands and fingers are now alternately used to strike the area more firmly (Fig 91).

Usage: As a stimulatory massage usually pre-competition and during the conditioning phase of training.

Effects: Hacking produces stimulation of local circulation depending upon the depth of application. If performed over certain areas it can provoke tendon and muscle reflexes (for example, patellar tendon – knee jerk). This manipulation will stimulate muscle tone and give a generalized feeling of stimulation.

Precautions: Usual contraindications apply. It is good practice to cover the skin area being treated with thin cloth to prevent skin irritation – do not use rough material such as towelling as this only irritates.

Clapping

Description of manipulation: The hands are held cupped and by alternately flexing and extending the wrists the area to be treated is struck by the hands.

Depth: Grade 1 – skin clapping; this manipulation is performed at a fast rate and quite lightly to produce skin stimulation. Grade 2 – muscle clapping; for this manipulation the rate of performance is slower and the strike firmer. Grade 3 – clapping; this evacuates hollow organs (such as the lungs) but is not often used in sports massage although it can be helpful in treating long-distance competitors suffering from chest problems at the end of events. The strike is very firm and the elbow as well as the wrist can be used to obtain a larger movement.

Performance: The hands are held with the fingers and thumbs in contact to form a cup shape (*see* practice on a pillow, Fig 10). Elbows are held away from the body and bent to about 90

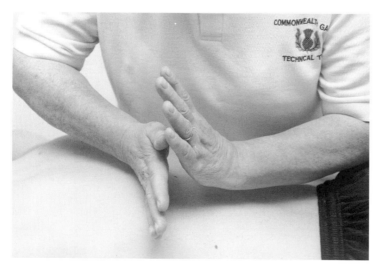

Fig 91. Grade 2 hacking, using outer border hands and fingers.

degrees. The wrists are alternately flexed and extended so that the cupped hands strike the skin and a hollow sound is produced (Fig 92).

Usage: Same as hacking.

Effects: Same as hacking but it has no effect on muscle or tendon reflexes.

Precautions: Usual contraindications apply. Ensure that the hands are not held too stiffly or the strike will produce pain. In grade 3 clapping, always cover the area being treated.

Beating

Description of manipulation: The hands are held in a loosely clenched fist and are used to hit the area by alternately flexing and extending the wrists.

Depth: Grade 1 is a fast rate, with fairly light contact to produce skin stimulation. Grade 2 is a slower rate with firmer contact to produce effects on muscle tissue. Grade 3 is mainly intended to evacuate hollow organs, but in sports massage it is used to help warm up exhausted long/ultra-distance competitors.

As in clapping, the strike is very firm and the area should be protected with cloth.

Performance: The hands are held in loosely clenched fists, with the thumbs held against the first finger (Fig 93). In grade 1 and 2 the wrists are flexed and extended to allow the fist to strike the area (Fig 94). In grade 3 the whole arm is raised and this allows the fist to be used for a strong, deep strike (Fig 95).

Usage: The use is as hacking, plus post competition as described above at grade 3.

Effects: These are as hacking but without an effect on reflexes and to induce a feeling of warmth.

Precautions: Usual contraindications apply. The hands must be relaxed on contact with the skin or manipulation will become too painful for the participant to tolerate. Always protect the skin with a cloth covering, especially when using grade 3.

Pounding

Description of manipulation: This is the same

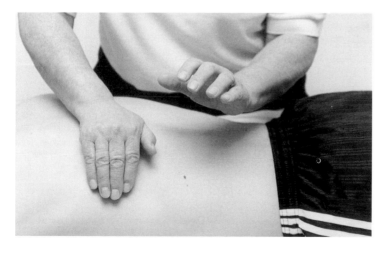

Fig 92. Clapping, wrist action and hand position.

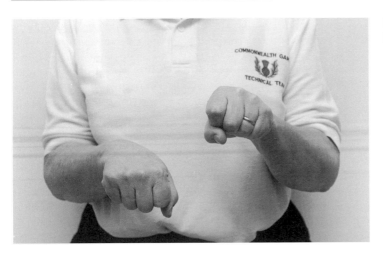

Fig 93. Beating, hand position.

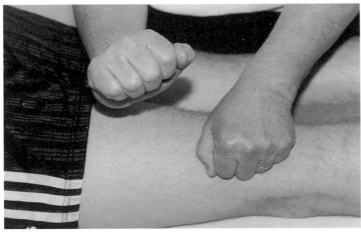

Fig 94. Grade 1 and 2 beating, wrist action.

action as hacking, but instead of using the whole hand, the hands are held in a loosely made fist and the contact takes place between the little finger and the area to be treated.

Depth: Grade 1 is at a fast rate, with light contact to stimulate skin. Grade 2 is a slower rate, with firmer contact to stimulate muscle. Grade 3 is as in beating to produce warmth and a feeling of well-being.

Performance: The hands are held in loosely clasped fists with the thumbs resting against the first fingers. The stance and start position

are as in hacking and contact is made with the little finger side of the fist (Fig 96).

Usage: The same as beating above.

Effects: The same as beating above.

Precautions: Usual contraindications apply, otherwise the precautions are as for beating.

Shaking

There are two categories of manipulation covered by this heading: shaking; and vibration.

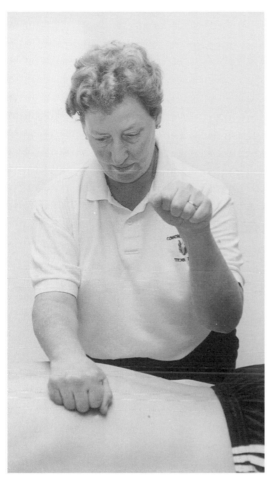

Fig 95. Grade 3 beating, whole arm action.

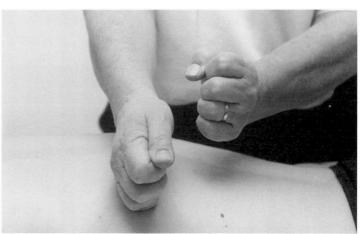

Fig 96. Pounding – contact with side of little finger.

Shaking

Description of manipulation: In skin and muscle shaking either the full length of the thumb and all the fingers are used to shake the tissue from side to side, or when treating smaller areas the tip of the thumb and one, two or three fingers are used to perform the shaking. In whole-limb shaking the leg or arm is lifted, gently supported and then shaken.

Depth: Grade 1 requires a very light application to stimulate superficial tissues. Grade 2 requires a firmer full grasp so that muscle tissue is lifted from underlying structures and then shaken. It affects deeper structures. Grade 3 applies to whole-limb shaking.

Performance: To perform grade 1 skin shaking the palm should not make contact – either the tip of the thumb and finger/fingers or whole thumb and all fingers are place on either side of the tissue (Figs 97 & 98). The hand is then rapidly shaken from side to side. For grade 2 the hand position is as 1 but a firmer grasp is applied and the shaking movement is repeated (Fig 99). For grade 3 the leg or arm is lifted and supported comfortably and then shaken (Fig 100).

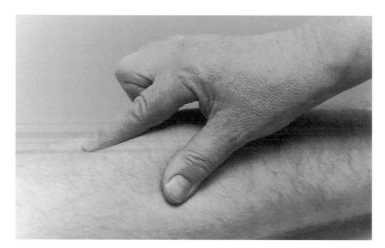

Fig 97. Grade 1 shaking, using tip of finger and thumb.

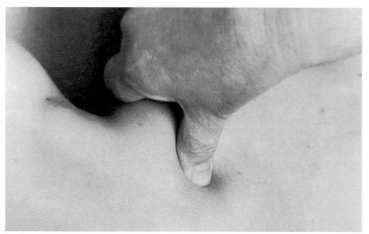

Fig 98. Grade 2 shaking, whole finger and thumb.

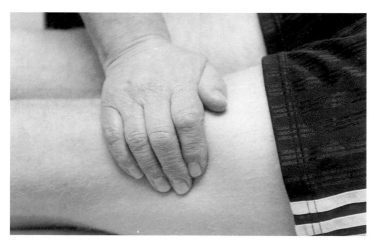

Fig 99. Grade 2 shaking, whole hand.

Usage: This technique can form part of a stimulating massage to relieve tension or can come at the end of a session prior to final effleurage.

Effects: It produces a feeling of stimulation and invigoration. It increases the mobility of tissues and helps to break down tissue adhesions. Shaking also stimulates venous and lymphatic flow and helps to prepare soft tissues for warm-up and stretch procedures.

Precautions: Usual contraindications apply. Care must be taken in grades 1 and 2 to ensure that the tissue is not nipped when the thumb and finger/s are applied. In grade 3 when the whole limb is shaken, the competitor must be relaxed and the limb shaken so as not to produce kickback on any joint or any feeling of strain.

Vibration

Description of manipulation: In this manipulation the tissues are pressed, moved up and down and then released. Either the whole hand or fingers only are used to perform the movement.

Depth: Grade 1 is a very light rapid movement to affect only superficial tissues. Grade 2 is a firmer, slower movement to move deeper structures and affect deeper structures. Grade 3 is as firm a pressure as can be tolerated by the participant, with a slow action that may compress tissue on underlying bone.

Performance: The manipulation is usually performed using one hand (Fig 101). If the competitor is large and the area to be treated is extensive two hands may be used (Fig 102). The masseur's arm should be positioned away from the body, with elbow slightly bent and fingers touching. The hand is then placed on the area to be treated, the tissue is compressed and the hand performs a forwards and backwards movement which causes the tissues to oscillate (Fig 103). In fingers-only application, the palm does not make contact and the fingers apply the movement.

Usage: As part of stimulating massage and to provide a feeling of well-being.

Effects: Vibration stimulates muscle tone and local circulation, while also providing a feeling of well-being.

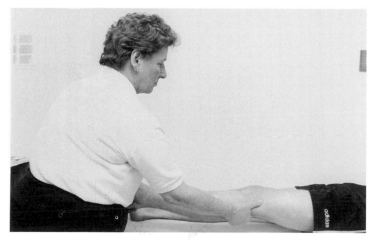

Fig 100. Grade 3 shaking, whole limb.

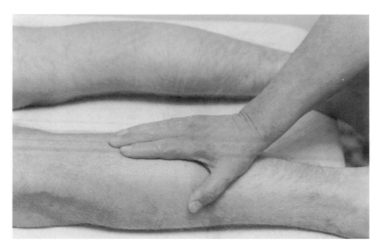

Fig 101. Vibration, one hand.

Fig 102. Vibration, two hands.

Precautions: Usual contraindications apply. Hand contact must be firm enough not to produce a ticklish sensation.

Acupressure and Trigger Pointing

The terms acupressure and trigger pointing are frequently used synonymously. However, this is not accurate and each manipulation must be recorded as a separate entity.

Acupressure

Description of the manipulation: Acupressure has come to the West from the East. To fully understand the origins and principles of acupressure the student must undertake a full study of the basic concepts of oriental medicine, which is not within the scope of this publication. For the purpose of sports massage, acupressure points are used to help eliminate stiff muscles, reduce specific pain in muscle tissues or joints, and to remove delayed onset muscle soreness. The technique involves pressing Tsubo or Shiatsu points, which are situated along a system of meridians (Figs 104, 105 & 106).

Depth: It is necessary to distinguish between

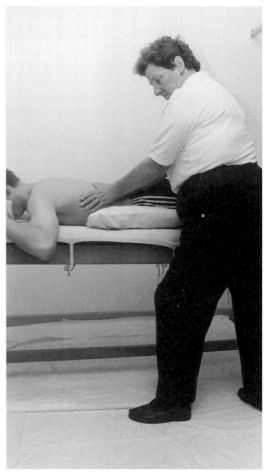

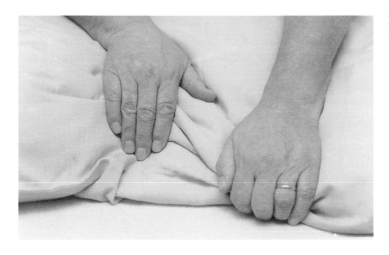

Fig 103. Vibration action, forward and backward.

Yin and Yang before addressing the depth of acupressure. Yin originally meant the shady side of the slope, associated with cold, rest, responsiveness, darkness and decrease. Yang originally referred to the sunny side of the slope and is associated with brightness, heat, stimulation, light and excitement. Yin and Yang are therefore complementary opposites. When Yin and Yang are balanced, the person should be in a state of good health and well-being; when they are out of balance ill health results.

If Yin is depleted, acupressure should be performed using slow gentle pressure along the direction of energy flow – this is grade 1. If Yang is depleted, acupressure should be performed more quickly with deeper pressure against the flow of energy – this is grade 2. There is no grade 3.

Performance: Acupressure is performed by application of thumb, fingertip, knuckle or elbow to the specific point to be influenced by the manipulation (Figs 107, 108, 109 & 110). Major acupressure points are illustrated in Figs 111, 112 and 113. The point is pressurized by the thumb, finger, knuckle or elbow; the small circular motion is described for a maximum of

two minutes. The recommended points on the affected side should be treated first and then the same points on the other side of the body. For localized complaints concentrate mainly on that side of the body.

Usage: Acupressure can be used as part of sports massage to reduce pain, to relax muscle tissue and promote a feeling of balance and good health.

Effects: Acupressure produces pain relief by release of endorphins, and stimulates local circulation and local lymph flow. It may be either stimulative or create relaxation depending upon which energy channel is used.

Precautions: Great caution is necessary when using acupressure points because of the possible effects on other structures. Acupressure should not be used on any person with heart disease or any known visceral condition. **Always be safe and ensure a full diagnosis by an appropriate professional**. Only fully trained and qualified practitioners should use acupressure for anything other than pain relief or muscle relaxation. Never use points LI4 (located in the web between the thumb and

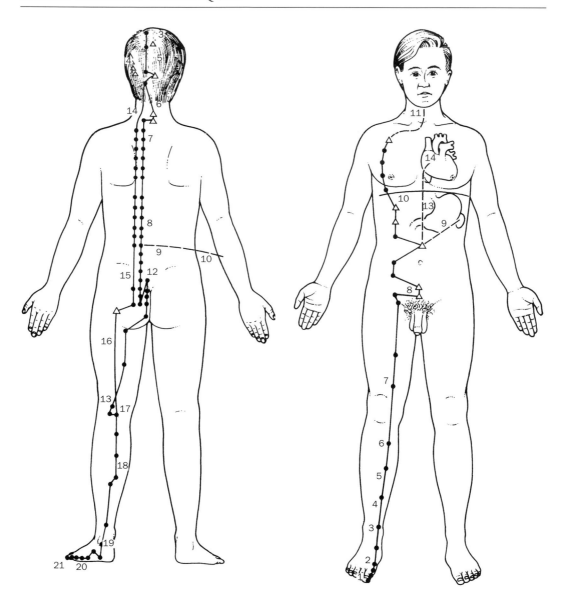

Fig 104. Meridians.

Fig 105. Meridians.

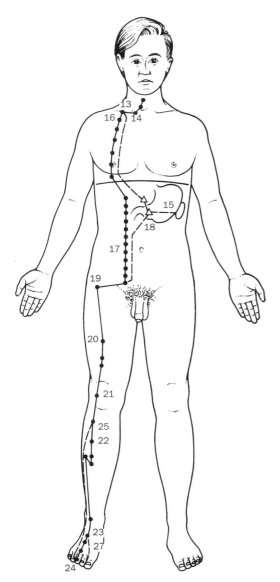

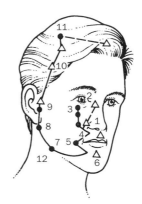

Fig 106. Meridians.

first finger on the back of the hand) or Sp6 (four finger widths above the medial malleolus, just behind the tibia) during pregnancy.

Trigger Pointing

Trigger points are narrow bands of fibres within a muscle which have been held in spasm or increased tone (Travell and Simons, 1992). Pressure of the point produces the pain, a distinct tight band is palpable and a twitch response is elicited when a finger slides over the tight band.

Description of the manipulation: A deep stroking is performed by the finger or thumb tip/s or direct pressure is applied to the trigger point by thumb, fingertip/s or elbow.

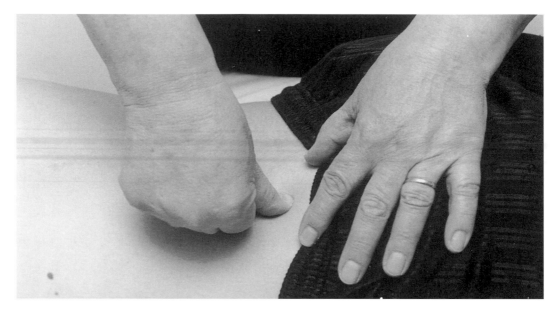

Fig 107. Acupressure, using thumbs.

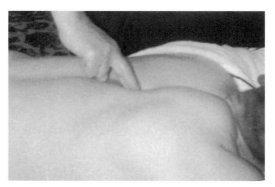

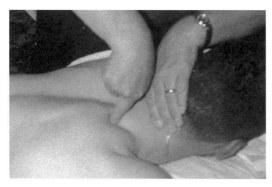

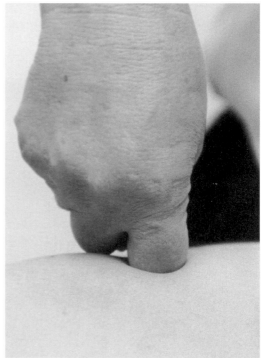

Fig 108. Acupressure, using fingertip.

Fig 109. Acupressure, using knuckle.

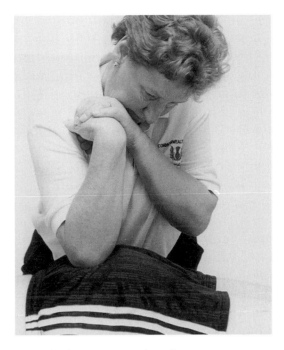

Fig 110. Acupressure, using elbow.

Depth: There is no grade 1. Grade 2 is a deep stroking to produce an effect on superficial tissues and vessels. Grade 3 is direct pressure, as much as the participant can tolerate, to produce effects on deep tissues and vessels.

Performance: Deep stroking performed by the fingertip or tips or by the thumb tip/s, along the full length of the affected fibres. It may be in any direction (Fig 114). Direct pressure is applied to the trigger point with the fingertip/s, thumb tip/s or elbow at 90 degrees to the tissue (Figs 115, 116, & 117). The pressure is maintained for 20 to 25 seconds, released and reapplied until relaxation is achieved.

Usage: This technique is used when the competitor reports specific tight areas and trigger points are identified. It is particularly useful pre- and inter-competition when time is limited and/or clothing cannot easily be removed.

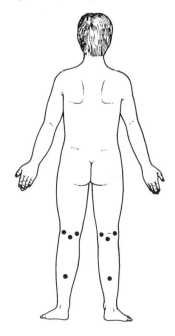
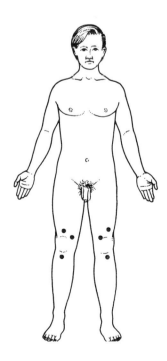

Fig 111. Major acupressure points.

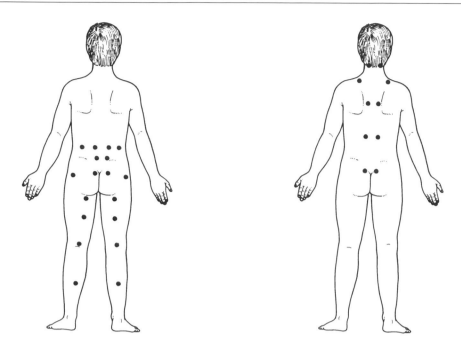

Fig 112. Major acupressure points.   Fig 113. Major acupressure points.

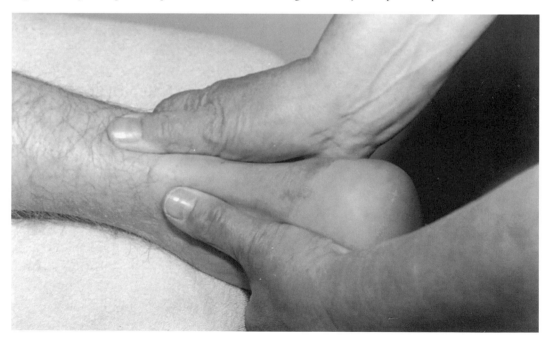

Fig 114. Trigger pointing.

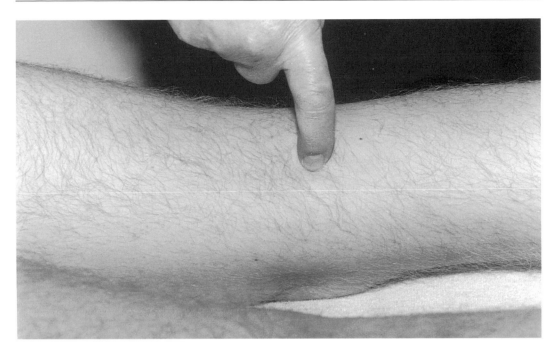

Fig 115. Trigger pointing with fingertip.

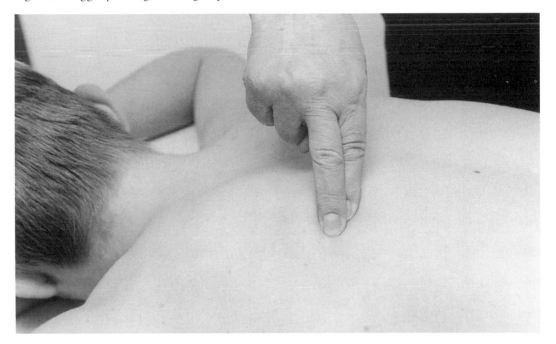

Fig 116. Trigger pointing with fingertips.

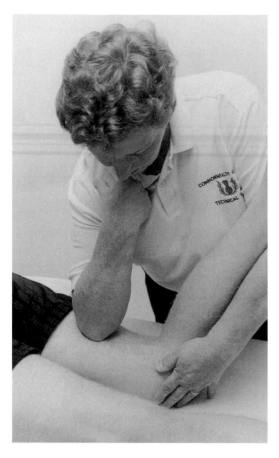

Fig 117. Trigger pointing with elbow.

Effects: It is effective for: pain relief; reduction of muscle spasm; helping muscle tone to return to normal; and allows the full stretch of tissues to occur. When full range has been gained the trigger point will no longer be active.

Precautions: The usual contraindications apply. Only use this technique on identified trigger points and follow it with full range stretching.

CHAPTER 4
Massage Terminology and Notation

The increase in the number of practitioners of massage and the fact that many sports participants now travel the world has made the usage of an understandable and recognizable language necessary. Practitioners who use various forms of manipulations, such as Maitland techniques, can notate their treatments and be understood by all other Maitland-trained therapists worldwide.

The following terminology and notation have been devised and used in an attempt to put all masseurs in a position where they can communicate meaningfully with their fellow practitioners. In no way is it meant to be prescriptive or to standardize the massage treatment.

STROKING MANIPULATIONS

Effleurage

Effleurage may be whole-handed centripetal, unidirectional, multi-directional, circular, figure seven, figure eight, or T-shaped. It may be performed with one hand, two hands, reinforced or with one, two or more fingers or the thumb.

Manipulation – Effleurage

- E = effleurage
- WH1 = whole hand one
- WH2 = whole hand two
- 1F = one finger
- 2F = two finger (three – 3F, four – 4F)
- 1T = one thumb (two – 2T)

The direction of manipulation can also be noted:

- ↑ = centripetal
- ↓ = centrifugal
- → = unidirectional to right
- ← = unidirectional to left
- M = multidirectional
- O = circular
- 7 = figure seven
- 8 = figure eight
- T = T-shaped

Depth may be:

- GR1 = grade 1
- GR2 = grade 2
- RE = reinforced

Examples of Notation

E WH2 7 GR2 is the notation for effleurage two-handed performed in a figure seven shape to grade 2 depth. E 2F→ GR1 is the notation for effleurage two fingers performed in unidirection to the right to grade 1 depth. All methods of applying effleurage can be recorded with application, direction and depth.

Stroking

Stroking may be grade 1 – single whole hand,

whole hand right then left, pad of finger, thumb or alternate, or thousand hands. Grade 2 can also use the ulnar surface of the fist, ulnar border of the palm, heel of the palm, ulnar border of the forearm, or the elbow as well as those noted for grade 1.

Manipulation – Stroking

- S = stroking
- WH1 = whole hand one (WH2 – whole hand two)
- WH R/L = whole hand right then left
- PF1 = pad of one finger
- PF2 = pads of two fingers (PF3 = three finger, PF4 = four fingers)
- PFT = pad of thumb
- TH = thousand hands
- USF = ulnar surface of fist
- UBP = ulnar border of palm
- HP = heel of palm
- UBF = ulnar border of forearm
- EL = elbow

The direction may be:

- ↑ = centripetal
- ↓ = centrifugal
- X = cross-over

Depth may be:

- GR1 = grade 1
- GR2 = grade 2

Examples of Notation

S WH1 ↑ GR2 is the notation for stroking whole hand one, centripetal (towards the heart) grade 2. S UBP2 X GR1 is the notation for stroking ulnar borders of both palms cross-over grade 1. S TH ↓ GR1 is the notation for stroking thousand hands centrifugal grade 1.

PRESSURE MANIPULATIONS OR PETRISSAGE

Kneading

Kneading may be palmar aspect of the whole hand, one, two, alternate or both. Finger kneading uses all fingers or combinations of one, two, three or four. Kneading also uses finger or thumb pad or tip of finger or thumb.

Manipulation – Kneading

- K = kneading
- WH1 and WH2 = whole hand one and two
- WH R/L = whole hand right then left alternate
- P = palm only
- FF1 = finger one (FF2 = fingers two, FF3 = fingers three, FF4 = fingers four)
- PF1 = pad of finger one (PT1 = pad of thumb one, PF3 = pads of three fingers, and so on)
- FT1 = finger tip one (TT = thumb tip, FT4 = four finger tips, and so on)

The direction may be:

- ↑ = centripetal
- ↓ = centrifugal

Depth may be:

- GR1 = grade 1
- GR2 = grade 2
- GR3 = grade 3 = reinforced

Examples of Notation

K WH2 ↑ GR3 is the notation for kneading two whole hands, centripetal reinforced grade 3. K FF4 ↓ GR1 is for full four fingers, centrifugal (away from the heart) grade 1.

Picking Up

Picking up can be single-handed C-shaped, double-handed C-shaped, single-handed V-shaped or double-handed V-shaped.

Manipulation – Picking Up

- PU = picking up
- WH1 = whole hand one (WH2 = whole hand two)
- C = C-shaped
- V = V-shaped

Direction may be:

- ↑ = centripetal
- ↓ = centrifugal
- → = to the right
- ← = to the left

Depth may be:

- GR1 = grade 1
- GR2 = grade 2
- GR3 = grade 3

Examples of Notation

PU WH2 C → GR2 is the notation for picking up two whole hands, C-shaped to the right, grade 2. PU WH1 V ↑ GR1 is the notation for picking up single whole hand, V-shaped, centripetal grade 1.

Wringing

Wringing can be performed by the fingers and thumbs or on larger areas by the whole hand.

Manipulation – Wringing

- W = wringing

- WH2 = whole-handed two (always use both hands)
- F/T = fingers and thumbs

Direction may be:

- ↑ = centripetal
- ↓ = centrifugal
- → = to the right
- ← = to the left
- M = multidirectional

Depth may be:

- GR1 = grade 1
- GR2 = grade 2

Examples of Notation

W F/T M GR1 is the notation for wringing using fingers and thumbs, multidirectional grade 1. W WH2 → GR2 is for wringing, using both hands to the right, grade 2.

Rolling

In this manipulation the whole of both hands is used as previously described.

Manipulation – Rolling

- R = rolling
- SK = skin, depth GR1 = grade 1
- M/S = muscle, depth GR2 = grade 2

Direction may be:

- ↑ = centripetal
- ↓ = centrifugal
- M = multidirectional

Examples of Notation

R SK GR1 M is the notation for skin rolling

grade 1 multidirectional. R M/S GR2 ↑ is the notation for muscle rolling grade 2 towards the heart.

FRICTIONS

Frictions may be circular friction or transverse friction.

Circular Friction

Manipulation – Circular Friction

- FS = friction
- F = finger
- T = thumb
- O = circular

Direction of circular friction is either clockwise to the right or anticlockwise to the left:

- → = to the right
- ← = to the left

Depth may be:

- GR2 = grade 2
- GR3 = grade 3

Examples of Notation

FS F O GR2 ← is the notation for friction with one finger, circular, grade 2 to the left. FS T O GR3 → is the notation for friction with the thumb, circular, grade 3 (reinforced) to the right.

Transverse Friction

Manipulation – Transverse Friction

In Cyriax training, transverse frictions are noted as DTF = deep transverse frictions.

DTF would be equivalent to grade 3 in this notation.

- FS = friction
- F = finger
- T = thumb
- TR = transverse

Direction may be:

- → = to the right
- ← = to the left

Depth is always GR3 = grade 3 (reinforced).

Examples of Notation

FS F TR GR3 → is the notation for friction with the finger, transverse, grade 3 to the right, as is FS F DTF → . FS T TR GR3 ← is the notation for friction with the thumb, transverse, grade 3 to the left, as is FS T DTF ←.

TAPOTEMENT

Hacking

Manipulation – Hacking

- T/H = tapotement hacking (TH stands for thousand hands in stroking)

Direction may be:

- ↑ = centripetal
- ↓ = centrifugal
- → = to the right
- ← = to the left
- M = multidirectional

Depth may be:

- GR1 = grade 1
- GR2 = grade 2
- GR3 = grade 3

Examples of Notation

T/H GR1 ↑ is the notation for hacking grade 1 centripetal. T/H GR3 ← is the notation for hacking grade 3 to the left.

Clapping

Manipulation – Clapping

- T/C = clapping

Direction may be:

- ↑ = centripetal
- ↓ = centrifugal
- → = to the right
- ← = to the left
- M = multidirectional

Depth may be:

- GR1 = grade 1
- GR2 = grade 2
- GR3 = grade 3

Examples of Notation

T/C GR2 M is the notation for clapping grade 2 multidirectional. T/C GR1 → is the notation for clapping grade 1 to the right.

Beating

Manipulation – Beating

- T/B = beating

Direction may be:

- ↑ = centripetal

- ↓ = centrifugal
- → = to the right
- ← = to the left
- M = multidirectional

Depth may be:

- GR1 = grade 1
- GR2 = grade 2
- GR3 = grade 3

Examples of Notation

T/B GR2 ↓ is the notation for beating grade 2 centrifugal. T/B GR1 ← is the notation for beating grade 1 to the left.

Pounding

Manipulation – Pounding

- T/P = pounding

Direction and grades are as for beating above.

Examples of Notation

T/P GR3 M is the notation for pounding grade 3 multidirectional. T/P GR1 → is the notation for pounding grade 1 to the right.

SHAKING

Shaking

Manipulation – Shaking

- SH = shaking
- 1F = one finger (2F = two fingers, and so on)
- T = thumb
- TT = tip of thumb

Direction may be:

- ↑ = centripetal
- ↓ = centrifugal
- → = to the right
- ← = to the left
- M = multidirectional

Note: Grade 3 whole-limb shaking will always be centripetal (towards the heart) so therefore no need to note direction.

Depth may be:

- GR1 = grade 1
- GR2 = grade 2
- GR3 = grade 3 (whole-limb shaking)

Examples of Notation

SH TT GR1 → is the notation for shaking with thumb tip grade 1 to the right. SH GR3 LEFT LEG is the notation for whole limb shaking left leg centripetal.

Vibration

Manipulation – Vibration

- V = vibration
- WH = whole hand (WH1 = whole hand one, WH2 = whole hand two)
- F = finger

Direction may be:

- → = to the right
- ← = to the left
- M = multidirectional

Depth may be:

- GR1 = grade 1
- GR2 = grade 2
- GR3 = grade 3

Examples of Notation

V GR1 WH2 → is the notation for vibration grade 1, using two hands to the right. V GR3 4F M is the notation for vibration grade 3 using four fingers multidirectional.

ACUPRESSURE AND TRIGGER POINTING

Acupressure

There is already a clear definition of acupressure meridians as shown in Figs 104, 105 & 106.
These points are recorded as follows:

- Lu = lung   proximal to distal
- LI = large intestine   distal to proximal
- St = stomach   proximal to distal
- Sp = spleen   distal to proximal
- H = heart   proximal to distal
- SI = small intestine   distal to proximal
- B = bladder   proximal to distal
- K = kidney   distal to proximal
- HP = heart protector proximal to distal
- TH = triple heater   distal to proximal
- GB = gall bladder   proximal to distal
- Liv = liver   distal to proximal

Acupressure points are located along the meridians and depending upon which pathway are numbered proximal to distally or distal to proximally (as noted above). The measurement used is the Cun – 1 Cun is the distance between the proximal and distal joint of the participant's middle finger (Fig 118); 3 Cun is the breadth of all four fingers, kept together, at the proximal finger joints (Fig 119).

Summary of Acupressure Points

Following is a summary of the acupressure points most often used in sports massage:

Lung:
- Lu 5 – location is in the elbow crease, lateral to the biceps tendon.
  Usage: neck, shoulder tension and specific muscular pain, as well as tennis elbow.

- Lu 7 – location is 1.5 Cun above the transverse wrist crease on the thumb side.
  Usage: pain or tension in the neck muscles.

- Lu 9 – location is at the lateral end of the transverse crease of the wrist, lateral to the radial artery (12 Cun below Lu 5).
  Usage: neck, shoulder tension, specific shoulder pain and wrist pain. Can also be used to revive a person who has fainted.

Large Intestine:
- LI4 – location is midpoint of the shaft of second metacarpal bone towards the thumb.
  Usage: neck, shoulder tension, supraspinatus tendonitis, subacromial bursitis, biceps tendonitis, pain or spasm of trapezius and wrist pain.

- LI5 – location is in the anatomical 'snuff box'.
  Usage: wrist pain.

- LI10 – location is 2 Cun below the elbow crease on the lateral aspect.
  Usage: tennis elbow.

- LI11 – location is with elbow flexed, point is in the depression at the lateral end of the elbow crease.
  Usage: supraspinatus tendonitis, subacromial bursitis and tennis elbow.

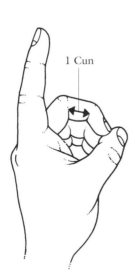

Fig 118. Measurement of 1 Cun.

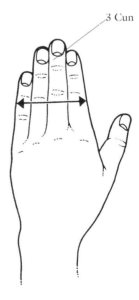

Fig 119. Measurement of 3 Cun.

- LI14 – location is at the deltoid insertion, on a line connecting LI11 and LI15.
  Usage: neck, shoulder syndrome, supraspinatus tendonitis, subacromial bursitis and tennis elbow.

- LI15 – location is shoulder abducted, the point is in the depression at the anterior border of the acromium.
  Usage: neck, shoulder syndrome, supraspinatus tendonitis.

- LI16 – location is in the dip between the acromial end of the clavicle and the spine of the scapula, medial to the acromio-clavicular joint.
  Usage: neck, shoulder syndrome, pain and spasm in the trapezius.

Stomach:
- St 34 – location is 2 Cun above the outer, upper border of the patella.
  Usage: knee pain.

- St 35 – location is with the knee flexed, the point is at the lower border of the patella in the dip lateral to the patellar tendon.
  Usage: anterior knee pain.

- St 36 – location is 0.5 Cun lateral to the tibial tubercle.
  Usage: general pain relief.

Spleen:
- Sp 6 – location is 3 Cun directly above the tip of the medial malleolus.
  Usage: ankle pain and shin pain.

- Sp 7 – location is 3 Cun above Sp 6, just behind the medial tibial border.
  Usage: shin pain.

- Sp 8 – location is 6 Cun below the lower patellar border, at the posterial tibial border.

Usage: shin pain.

- Sp 9 – location is in the dip on the lower border of the medial tibial condyle, level with the tibial tuberosity.
  Usage: localized knee-joint pain.

Heart:
- H3 – location is between the medial end of the elbow crease and the medial epicondyle with the elbow bent.
  Usage: tennis elbow.

- H5 – location is 1 Cun above the dip on the ulnar aspect, radial side of the wrist.
  Usage: wrist pain.

- H7 – location is on the ulnar side of the wrist in the dip.
  Usage: wrist pain.

Small Intestine:
- SI11 – location is in the infrascapular fossa in the dip in the centre.
  Usage: thoracic, shoulder and neck pain.

- SI12 – location is in the suprascapular fossa, directly above SI11.
  Usage: pain and spasm in the trapezius.

- SI15 – location is on the ulnar side of the wrist in the dip between the styloid of the ulna and the pisiform.
  Usage: wrist pain.

- SI16 – with the elbow bent and palm on the chest, the point is located in the bony cleft on the radial aspect of the ulnar styloid.
  Usage: wrist pain, pain and stiff joints in the arm and neck.

- SI18 – with the elbow bent, the point is located in the groove between the ole-

cranon and the medial epicondyle of the humerus.
Usage: golfer's elbow.

Bladder:
- B11 – location is 1.5 Cun lateral to the lower border of the T1 process.
  Usage: mid-thorax, shoulder or neck pain.

- B22 – location is 1.2 Cun lateral to the lower border of the L1 spinous process.
  Usage: low back pain, fatigue.

- B23 – location is 1.5 Cun lateral to the lower border of the L2 spinous process.
  Usage: low back pain, hamstring pain, sciatica.

- B25 – location is 1.2 Cun lateral to the lower border of the L4 spinous process.
  Usage: low back pain, sciatica.

- B50 – location is 3 Cun lateral to the lower border of the T12 spinous process.
  Usage: Hip pain, jogger's hip syndrome.

- B53 – location is 3 Cun lateral to the midline of the trunk, level with the S2 foramen.
  Usage: knee pain.

- B54 – location is 3 Cun lateral to the midline of the trunk level with the S4 foramen.
  Usage: knee pain.

- B57 – location is 8 Cun below the middle of the popliteal crease.
  Usage: muscle spasm in legs, and ankle or foot pain.

- B60 – location is in the dip between the lateral malleolus and the tendo-achilles (TA).
  Usage: hip syndromes, low back pain, sciatica, Achilles tendinitis.

Kidney:
- K3 – location is midway between the tip of the medial malleolus and TA.
  Usage: ankle pain, Achilles problems.

- K4 – location is behind and below K3 in the dip anterior to the insertion of the TA.
  Usage: ankle, foot, Achilles pain.

- K7 – location is 2 Cun above K3 on the anterior border of the TA.
  Usage: calf pain or spasm.

- K10 – with the knee bent, the point is located at the medial end of the popliteal crease.
  Usage: knee pain.

Note: Heart protector and triple heater points do not tend to be used in sports massage.

Gall Bladder:
- GB21 – location is the midpoint of a line connecting the acromium and the lower border of the C7 spinous process.
  Usage: stiff neck, shoulder and upper thoracic pain.

- GB25 – location is on the lateral side of the abdomen, at the lower end of the twelfth rib.
  Usage: rib, chest pain.

- GB29 – location is the midpoint between the line connecting the anterior superior iliac spine and the highest point of the greater trochanter.
  Usage: hip pain, gluteal pain.

- GB30 – location is in the dip lateral to the greater trochanter.
  Usage: hip, low back pain, sciatica.

- GB31 – location is 7 Cun above the transverse popliteal crease, on the lateral border

of the thigh where the middle finger touches when standing.
Usage: general aches and pains in the legs and hip pain.

- GB34 – location is in the dip anterior and inferior to the head of the fibula.
Usage: ankle and knee pain, and influences muscles and tendons anywhere in the body.

- GB41 – location is in the dip distal to the junction of the bases of the fourth and fifth metatarsals.
Usage: plantar fasciitis.

Liver:
- Liv 3 – location is in the dip distal to the bases of first and second metatarsals.
Usage: plantar fasciitis.

- Liv 5 – location is 5 Cun above the tip of the medial melleolus on the medial tibial border.
Usage: shin pain, 'shin splints'.

- Liv 8 – location is the medial end of the transverse crease of the knee joint.
Usage: knee pain, ITT syndrome.

Examples of Notation

ACU GB30 LEFT is the notation for acupressure gall bladder point 30 on the left. ACU H5, SI6 RIGHT AND LEFT is the notation for acupressure heart point 5 and small intestine point 6 right and left.

Trigger Pointing

Manipulation

- TR/P = trigger pointing
- F = finger (2F = two fingers, and so on)
- T = thumb
- FT = fingertip
- TT = thumb tip
- EL = elbow

Direction may be:

- ↑ = centripetal
- ↓ = centrifugal
- → = to the right
- ← = to the left
- M = multidirectional

Depth may be:

- GR2 = grade 2
- GR3 = grade 3

Examples of Notation

TR/P TT GR3M is the notation for trigger pointing with thumb tip grade 3 multidirectional. TR/P 4F GR2 ↑ is the notation for trigger pointing with four fingers grade 2 towards the heart.

The only other information which can be helpful to note is the length of time spent performing a massage. This will be addressed in detail in the description of massage usage.

CHAPTER 5
Sports Massage Application

Sports massage can be divided into two distinct areas of application:

1. Specific sports massage.
2. Non-specific sports massage.

SPECIFIC SPORTS MASSAGE

This heading covers sports massage used for a specific reason or purpose and can be applied to six different situations:

1. Massage in conditioning.
2. Massage as treatment.
3. Massage pre-competition.
4. Massage inter-competition.
5. Massage post-competition.
6. Massage post-travel.

Massage in Conditioning

The conditioning time of year for any sportsperson will depend entirely upon when their competitive season occurs and on their specific 'goals' for that year. The actual time of year when conditioning takes place will vary from sport to sport, dependent on competitive season and the timetables of major events. Each year must be examined individually to plan which events are major and will be targeted by the competitor and coach. It is accepted practice for sports coaches and scientists to plan in

four-year cycles, with the culmination being the Olympic games, world championships or similar high-profile events.

It is not unusual to have a major event in January and then another in August. If there is to be more than one major event in twelve months, then more than one peak of condition must be attained and conditioning times will differ from a one-only peak season. For example, 'peaking' for Olympic Team selection in June and then again to compete in the Olympic Games in September is very different to peaking once to compete in July. A principle often used is the 'SAID principle', Specific Adaptation Imposed Demands, as recorded by Walls and Logan. This principle puts the body through safe and intense development, to achieve peak condition at the time of the major competition. Massage during the conditioning phase of the sportsperson's year plays a very important part in the training regime.

Objectives of Massage in Conditioning

To promote faster recovery from a hard training session: It is to be expected after a hard bout of training and exercise that the sportsperson will experience various aches, pains and a feeling of tired, heavy limbs. Massage can be invaluable in speeding up recovery at this time and also allow sufficient recovery to permit a further training stint to take place in a shorter time. It can be possible to fit in at least two sessions per day, with massage being used as part of the recovery process

To aid cool-down: The object of cool-down is to return the body to its pre-exercise resting state as efficiently and painlessly as possible. Massage can be used at this time, before active cool-down and immediately after this activity. The main object of this form of sports massage is to promote circulation and lymphatic drainage. Massage will also assist in the removal of waste products and enable the participants to perform their own cool-down regimes more effectively.

To help in the improvement of mobility and flexibility: One of the most important activities during the time of conditioning must be to maintain and if possible increase the mobility and flexibility of the participant. This is particularly important when the conditioning period involves a lot of strength, endurance and stamina training. Flexibility is one of the most repetitive parts of training and probably the part most often skimped on or even totally missed out. However, the participant will be only too pleased to come for a massage. The main object of any massage aimed at enhancing flexibility must be to ensure an increase in circulation and soft-tissue mobility. As well as the strokes previously described, there are more advanced techniques used to enhance flexibility such as proprioceptive neuromuscular facilitation (PNF), passive and active stretching, neuromuscular techniques (NMT), muscle energy techniques (MET), soft tissue release (STR) and connective tissue massage (CTM). These are advanced manipulative techniques and should only be applied by adequately trained practitioners.

To prevent delayed onset muscle soreness (DOMS): It is widely accepted that intense bouts of exercise will produce degrees of muscle/soft tissue soreness after the event, especially if greater ranges of movement are being sought or greater levels of strength and stamina are being used. The soreness may not be noticed for up to 24 hours after cessation of the activity. Many learned sources will insist that there is no scientific proof that massage will in any way prevent the occurrence of DOMS. On the other hand, observation and anecdotal evidence leads those who are actively engaged in the field of sports massage to feel sure that DOMS can be influenced positively by the application of the correct massage techniques. The main object in the prevention of DOMS is to increase circulation, stimulate lymphatic drainage, separate tissues, identify muscle/soft tissue tension and promote relaxation.

Psychological effect: The importance of the psychological effect of touch has never been fully quantified. Only in more recent times has it been awarded its place in the effects of massage and it should never be underestimated. During the conditioning time of sport, the participant is working extremely hard, frequently under the guidance of one person – the coach. It is very easy for tempers to flare and little problems to be magnified out of all proportion. A visit to a masseur, away from the coach, other competitors and the frustrations of repetitive activities can be invaluable in restoring the equilibrium. Massage delivered by a good, knowledgeable practitioner can make a vast difference to the participant's continued well-being and enhance the positive effects of the conditioning phase. The object of this massage will either be stimulatory or relaxing, depending upon the requirements of that particular time of conditioning. If conditioning is still ongoing or between activities, stimulation will be required. If the day, block of activity or full conditioning has ended, relaxation will be best.

Contact Materials to be Used in Conditioning Massage

Oil-based media are preferred in this form of massage as good contact is required. Frequently the conditioning phase will take place at a training camp which may well be situated in a warm/hot climate. This environment will immediately rule out several massage media, such as hot rubs or powders. In hot climates warming/hot rubs are most uncomfortable, producing too much increase in superficial circulation which, as well as being unpleasant, interferes with the body's cooling mechanism. Powder also tends to clog the skin pores and can create too much friction on perspiring skin. It is important that the participant is happy with the massage medium being used and you should always ascertain what their particular preference is. However, if they ask for a hot rub be sure there are no contraindications to its application, such as micro-trauma after a hard training session. Also ensure that the participant is aware of the reaction to a hot rub when applied in a hot country. In colder climates it may well be beneficial to finish the massage with the use of a mild warming agent.

It is usually possible for the participant to have cleansed the skin before massage in the conditioning period and also to be able to shower or bathe immediately after the massage. Warm soapy water as a massage medium is extremely acceptable at this stage and also cuts down on post-massage cleansing. You should also bear in mind that if the skin is exposed to more than usual sunlight there may be a delayed reaction, and it is always wise to ensure that all participants are aware of sensible sun exposure.

Techniques Used in Conditioning Massage

Stroking grade 1 (GR1), followed by grade 2

(GR2) and effleurage grade 3 (GR3): Accustoms the participant to the masseur's touch; clears the drainage pathways towards the lymph glands, and allows the masseur to identify any tight, tense areas or area of micro-trauma after a hard training session.

- *Effleurage GR2:* Promotes venous and lymphatic drainage.

Petrissage starting with GR1 and increasing to GR3 as applicable: All techniques in petrissage may be utilized. This will increase the mobility of tissues, help with the removal of waste products, and increase the length and strength of connective tissues.

- *Effleurage GR2:* Promotes venous and lymphatic drainage.

Acupressure: Apply to any specific points of tension identified.

Trigger pointing: Apply as needed to any identified trigger spots.

Stroking GR2: Provides relaxation and aids venous return.

Tapotement/shaking vibrations: All of these techniques or a choice of one or more can be carried out to GR2 to produce stimulation and a feeling of well-being.

- *Effleurage GR2 down to GR1:* To aid venous, lymphatic return, ensure there is no congestion in the tissues, and assess the final state of the tissues.

Method of Application of Conditioning Massage

If applying full body massage at the end of a training day or at the end of a conditioning session, start with the back, then the limbs and anterior torso. Concentrate on the muscles most used and those exhibiting most tension. It is often very useful to finish with a relaxing foot massage.

Sometimes the massage will be applied between training sessions and in that case requirements must be identified whether to stimulate, relax, remove waste products or aid flexibility. Once the reason has been established then the area/areas needing attention should be addressed.

Duration of Conditioning Massage

Whole-body massage will last 1 to 1½ hours. Half-body will last ½ to ¾ of an hour. Any specific area should be addressed as needed until the desired effect has been obtained. Massage can be given on a daily basis throughout the conditioning phase. The first massage should be given the day before the start of the conditioning to enable the masseur to recognize any old/long-standing damage areas, any particular tension areas and to get the 'feel' of the participant's tissue when relaxed.

Contraindications to Conditioning Massage

All contraindications as already listed in Chapter 2 will apply. Pay particular attention to ensuring that any micro-trauma that may have been occasioned by hard training is avoided when applying all massage techniques – **if in doubt seek the correct professional help**.

Massage as Treatment

Sports injury may be treated with massage after 48 hours if all bleeding and tissue swelling has ceased. In the case of haematoma, massage can be used after four days or dependent upon the competitor's tolerance. The initial diagnosis and referral for massage must come from the appropriate professional, either a doctor or physiotherapist.

Objectives of Massage as Treatment

To stimulate circulation: 48 hours after soft tissue trauma it is vital to clear away the debris of the incident and remove excess tissue fluid. Massage can play an important part in attaining these goals. The main object of this massage is to clear the blood vessels and lymph vessels around the area of damage, and in particular to address any area of congestion or stagnation and encourage good flow to and from the damaged part. In the case of haematoma it is particularly important to ensure that there is no congestion impeding the venous return from the area of trauma.

To promote recovery from injury: The better the blood supply to an area, the better the recovery. The object of this massage is to promote the blood supply to and from the specific damaged area and so give a better base for recovery. Holey and Cook state that 'Remodelling of connective tissue during the healing process can be facilitated by massage'.

To break down adhesions: It is vitally important after injury in sport that the participant has not been left with a tight, shortened scar in any soft tissue. The presence of adhesion and scar tissue are sources of further trauma and under stresses of training, especially stretching and flexibility, can break down. This may cause re-injury with resultant bigger scar areas. The object of massage in this instance is again to promote circulation and also to mobilize the soft tissues and release adherent tissues.

To promote flexibility: It is essential that all sports people maintain their levels of flexibility during recovery from injury. Before a return to training and competition the level of movement and flexibility of the injured part must be equal to that of the non-injured opposite limb or at the same level as was attainable prior to the injury. The object of massage in this instance is to enable the tissues surrounding the injury to maintain their maximum potential for stretch during the early healing phase. As the recovery proceeds the massage can encroach more and more onto the healing area and promote the stretch of that tissue.

To improve the range of movement: Unfortunately, most types of injury, both soft-tissue and bony, may well necessitate periods of immobilization, with strapping, plaster or splints. As with flexibility, it is essential to have full-range movement prior to a return to full training and competition. The object of massage here is to help reduce tissue tone, promote circulation and facilitate full-range joint movements.

Psychological effect: Again, as previously stated, this aspect of massage should not be negated and in recovery from injury the masseur can play an important part by keeping accurate records to demonstrate the gains. Measurements to demonstrate reduction of swelling, increase in flexibility and movement are all very helpful in the psychology of injury recovery.

Contact Materials to be Used in Massage as Treatment

There are numerous lubricants which can be used in this form of massage, such as oils, creams, heat rubs (again, there is nothing to be gained by using a very hot rub), anti-inflammatory gel or cream and preparations such as Arnica. Frequently used are water alone or with soap, ice massage and various essential oils (both to be dealt with in a later chapter). A light talcum powder is also useful and some participants prefer this to oily preparations. As before, consider the competitor's preferences and as long as these are not contraindicated or negate the massage objects, try to accommodate any requests. It should be remembered that a much greater depth can be attained in massage when no lubricant is used.

Techniques Used in Massage as Treatment

Stroking GR 1 followed by GR 2: This accustoms the participant to the masseur's touch, clears the drainage pathways, and discovers any areas of sensitivity. At a first session after injury this may be all that can be tolerated and should only be applied distal and proximal to the actual site of injury.

- *Effleurage:* The depth will depend on the injury status, early GR1 only advancing to GR3 as recovery takes place – and is used to promote venous and lymphatic drainage. It can also be interspersed between more aggressive techniques to produce relaxation.

Petrissage: Again starting with GR1 up to GR3 as required and/or tolerated, using all techniques. The aim is to mobilize soft tissues, induce a slight stretch reflex, reduce muscle spasm and increase the strength and length of the connective tissues.

- *Effleurage:* as stated above.

Transverse frictions: Performed to GR3, as the participant can tolerate, to produce a local increase in circulation to aid the removal of inflammation. This technique has also a counter-irritant effect to reduce pain, stretches fibrous tissues, mobilizes the soft tissues, and separates adherent tissues.

- *Effleurage:* GR1 to GR2 should always follow transverse frictions to remove the possibility of any congestion in the treatment area, and to promote relaxation.

Tapotement: A selection of techniques as applicable and acceptable to the participant to GR2 in order to promote excitation in the tissue, and produce a feeling of well-being.

- *Effleurage:* as above.

Shaking: GR1 and GR2 applied locally, to aid relaxation and relieve muscle tension and cramp. If done to GR3, total limb shaking, promotes relaxation.

Rolling: GR2, applied to affected area, mobilizes scar tissues.

- *Effleurage:* GR2 down to GR1 aids venous and lymphatic return, ensures no congestion remains in the area of treatment and assesses the final state of the treatment area.

Method of Application of Treatment Massage

Always start massage proximal then distal to the area to be treated, so as to ensure open channels of drainage. Gradually encroach onto the specific area of damage within the participant's toleration level. If providing another form of massage to another body area, perform the treatment massage first and allow a follow up for final observations of any post-treatment reactions.

Duration of Treatment Massage

Duration is totally dependent upon the state and sensitivity of the area to be treated. It may last from 10 minutes up to 30 minutes. The treatment can be used frequently during the day, once daily, or may require rest days depending upon the reaction level, the participant's discomfort and their training/competition schedule.

Contraindications to Treatment Massage

All contraindications as previously indicated will apply. **Accurate diagnosis and prognosis must be obtained from a suitably qualified person**. Never apply if the participant can not tolerate the treatment, and do not use within three days of training or competition if the methods are aimed at treating scar tissue or adhesions. **Warning: always advise participant of any possible reaction and recommend the use of ice packs**.

Massage Pre-Competition

Massage prior to training and competition is to many sports people an essential part of the preparation ritual, the timing of which has to be carefully planned. For example, if one masseur has to deal with a team sport and all the players require a massage, there could be twenty or more massages to be performed. There must therefore be adequate staff available so that pre-competition massages do not have to be given many hours before the actual physical warm-up. In the case of an individual performance, the report time and/or start time will dictate the time of the pre-competition massage: for example, start time 11am, report time 10.40am, warm-up one hour, so the pre-competition massage must start at 9.10am at the latest. A rushed pre-competition massage is not performed well and will not help the participant's performance.

Warm-Up

Warm-up is the term used to denote the preparation of the body for physical activity. It is divided into three components:

1. Raising body temperature and increasing cardiovascular activity.
2. Putting all joints through the fullest range of movement available to them and all muscles into their greatest length of flexibility.
3. Sport-specific warm-up by mimicking and practising the activities to be performed.

Raising body temperature and increasing cardiovascular activity: This is the first part of any warm-up programme and is dependent upon the duration of the warm-up and the ambient temperature. It will be a necessity to intersperse mobility and flexibility with further temperature activity. The temperature may be raised by jogging, cycling, skipping, pattering (similar to running on the spot without the toes ever breaking ground contact), or when dealing with the older, purely recreational participants, by standing up and sitting down on a chair.

Joint mobility and muscle flexibility: This should start at the neck and work downwards to the feet or from the feet up to the neck. Each joint and each muscle group should be put through a full range/extent of motion, with the position being held for a minimum of 15 seconds. If the warm-up is being performed outdoors or in a cold hall the stretches will be interspersed with activity to maintain body temperature and cardiovascular activity.

Sport-specific warm-up: This will consist of a mimic of all the patterns and activities to be performed. For example, a thrower will throw, a racquet player will have practice shots or shadow play, a hurdler will hurdle and a footballer will kick the ball. Pre-competition massage cannot replace and must never be used instead of the participant's own physical warm-up. However, this massage can be used to assist the individual's warm-up and will definitely enhance the effects of the activity.

Objectives of Pre-Competition Massage

To prepare muscles for activity and extremes of exertion: The main objective of this massage is to increase the circulation to all areas of the body and in particular to the specific muscle areas which are most used in the activity. Massage prior to the stretch exercises will make it easier to perform the specific movement necessary to increase flexibility.

To aid the effects of the physical activity of the warm-up: As the term implies, warm-up is about warming the body prior to activity. The vasodilatation produced by massage will enhance the effect of this physical preparation.

To promote flexibility: As previously stated in Massage as Treatment (*see* pages 84–6), massage prior to activity enables full stretch to be more easily reached.

To improve the range of movement: Again, as previously stated, the massage will facilitate the full range of joint movements.

Psychological effect: The time spent on the massage couch is a very important aspect of the pre-competition routine – many top class sports people would never dream of competing without this massage. Mental preparation for the forthcoming action can take place while the massage is being performed. This may be done in conversation with the masseur or may be inward and silent. Obviously there is a great advantage if the masseur and participant know one another well. The masseur then appreciates whether or not the participant likes to talk at this stage and also understands the individual preparation foibles. It is also a good time to reinforce positive messages and allay fears about injury worries and the state of the opposition.

Contact Materials to be Used in Pre-Competition Massage

In the pre-competition massage the lubricants to be used must be carefully selected, dependent upon the activity about to take place. Again, the climate and temperature must be taken into account. Oils, creams and light talcum are all appropriate, but do not use any heating agent. All heating creams/rubs will encourage vasodilatation of the skin and this will prove detrimental to the warm-up. Vasodilatation needs to be greatest below the dermis to provide the best aid to a warm-up. Superficial vasodilatation is also detrimental to the skin's cooling process. **It is vital that all traces of oil and cream are removed from the participant's skin at the end of the massage**. For example, oil left on a basketball player's thigh can easily be transferred to his hands with disastrous results for his ball-catching ability. Likewise, oil or cream left on the body of a long or triple jumper quickly attracts sand and can create horrific irritations.

Techniques Used in Pre-Competition Massage

Stroking GR1 followed by GR2 and effleurage GRI: This sequence accustoms the participant to touch, promotes venous and lymphatic return, identifies any particular tight or tense area and identifies any area of pain.

Petrissage: starting with GR1 and increasing to GR3 as the participant desires, all techniques of petrissage may be utilized. It increases the mobility of tissues, and increases the length and strength of connective tissues.

Tapotement: All of these techniques can be used, or one or two, to promote a feeling of well-being and to relieve muscle tension.

Effleurage GR2: This can be interspersed with and used to finish the massage so as to stimulate circulation and ascertain the final tissue state.

Trigger pointing and/or acupressure: These may have to be used if there are specific areas of spasm, tension or increased tone in order to produce as much flexibility in the tissue as possible.

Method of Application of Pre-Competition Massage

The most important person at this stage in the proceedings is the competitor. A pre-competition massage must be tailored to each individual competitor's requirements. Some may want a full-body massage, others may only require specific areas, such as hamstrings or calf muscles to be massaged. It may be that a participant wants only a few minutes of acupressure or trigger pointing – in fact, that may be all there is time to do. This is not the correct time or place to try to educate the participant on the finer points and niceties of massage – just deliver what is requested, providing that there are no contraindications. Save the lectures for another time.

Duration of Pre-Competition Massage

This depends on the body area to be massaged and the length of time required to achieve the desired effect of stimulation and to decrease any spasm or increased tone. Most frequently, pre-competition massage lasts for 20 to 30 minutes, but on occasions may be up to an hour. As a last minute aid to decrease specific muscle tensions, acupressure and trigger pointing may be applied for just a few minutes. If the masseur is versed in the techniques, soft tissue release and various muscle stretches or PNF can be extremely useful.

Contraindications to Pre-Competition Massage

All contraindications as previously listed will apply. It is most important never to use a hot rub, nor to massage undiagnosed problems. In addition, don't use massage for the first time in the pre-competition situation if the participant has not had massage on previous occasions.

Massage Inter-Competition

During competitions which have several rounds, such as qualifying, quarter-final, semi-final and perhaps even finals on the same day, there are periods of rest in-between. This is when massage can be very useful to the participant and help to relieve excess tiredness due to repetitive warm-up and cool-down. In track-and-field athletics, where the multi-events require the men to participate in ten events in two days and the women in seven, properly executed warm-up and cool-down would take too long and leave the competitor utterly exhausted. Massage is extremely useful in such circumstances to facilitate a shorter warm-up and cool-down, but again it must be remembered that massage cannot replace these essential activities.

Objectives of Inter-Competition Massage

To promote recovery: After a bout of exertion waste products will have built up in the tissues. The drainage pathways may well be overloaded and muscle actions could be lethargic. The main object of massage at this time is to stimulate circulation, improve drainage and help to restore the tissues to the pre-activity state.

To refresh the competitor: During prolonged competition it is not unusual to experience muscle fatigue and general tiredness. As the day progresses it becomes more and more difficult to keep motivated (especially if results are not going well) and approach the next stage of the competition phase with the correct attitude. Massage at this point can be used to produce stimulation and enhance a general feeling of well-being.

To work out 'niggles' and identify injury or possible injury: After repetitive bouts of hard exercise it is usual to find that some muscular areas feel tight or tense. The usual pattern of stretch exercises only seems to increase this tension and can make the participant fear the worst, that there is an injury. Frequently these tight, tense areas are muscle fibres which are holding slightly too much tone, and attempts to exercise it off only increase the problem. Massage at this stage can be used physically to reassure the participant that there is not a major injury worry. If there is any doubt about an area being the site of an injury or possible further trouble the participant should immediately be referred to the doctor or physiotherapist.

To prevent muscle cramps, spasms and DOMS: It is well recognized that cramps are adversely affected by dehydration. Whilst the participant is rehydrating, massage can be applied to help stimulate circulation to the extremities and so reduce cramps. DOMS, as previously noted, can be reduced by the application of massage.

Psychological effect: The inter-competition time can be extremely fraught for several reasons. The participant may not be performing as well as anticipated, their biggest rival may just have beaten them, or a personal best in the last event may have left them euphoric and with unrealistic expectations. The time spent on the masseur's couch is a private one between participant and masseur and can often be very important to the psychology involved in that sport. Obviously everyone benefits from a good rapport between the masseur, participant, coach and other team members. It is important when administering inter-competition massage to try to let the participant leave the couch with no extra 'hang-ups' produced by the wrong application of techniques or a thoughtless remark.

Contact Materials to be Used in Inter-Competition Massage

As in pre-competition massage the wrong lubricant can produce disastrous results. The first necessity may well be to clean the skin areas to be massaged. The chances are that this type of massage is to be administered either in a sports stadium or perhaps outdoors. It is highly unlikely that there will be the facility to shower, time to do so or even a desire on the part of the participant to do so. Wet/moist tissues are great for cleaning small areas but to deal with larger areas a spray bottle filled with either water or a mixture of water and liquid soap is better.

When the area has been cleaned, oil or light creams are the best choice of lubrication for massage. Do not use hot rubs as this will create too much superficial vasodilatation. Do not use talcum as this can inhibit the skin's facility to cool the body. Always ensure that all the massage lubricant has been removed at the end of the massage session. If appropriate, ensure that sun protection is reapplied before the participant goes out.

Techniques used in Inter-Competition Massage

Immediately after activity:

Stroking GR1, followed by GR2: This accus-

toms the participant to touch, which is very important to assess the temperature and general state of the skin and areas to be massaged. Remember that if there is no perspiration on the skin after strenuous activity the participant is probably severely dehydrated.

- *Effleurage GR1:* This will discover any particularly tense areas, pain or spasm, and also improve drainage, both venous and lymphatic.

Petrissage: Use a combination of all techniques to the depth that can be tolerated and be aware of any risk or potential damage.

- *Effleurage:* Perform to increasing depth if the participant feels happy with this.

Acupressure: Apply to any area which is identified as excessively tense or tending to cramp.

Trigger pointing: Apply to trigger points if this is tolerable to the participant.

- *Effleurage GR1:* Perform this to end the massage.

Immediately prior to active warm-up for next activity;

All techniques as described above plus:

Vibration GR3 M: This is very good to improve muscle stretch.

Shaking GR3 (whole limb): This is useful to stimulate and release any cramps.

Tapotement GR2: This will stimulate and provide a feeling of well-being.

- *Effleurage:* To be performed as deep as the participant requires.

Method of Application of Inter-Competition Massage

Early on the day the participant may wish only specific areas to be massaged, such as hamstring or calf muscles. As the competition proceeds the areas to be massaged are quite likely to become more extensive. It is often necessary to address most of the body after the penultimate event to give a help to cool-down and then repeat as a stimulation prior to the final warm-up activity.

Duration of Inter-Competition Massage

The simplistic statement to answer this is: as time allows. Realistically, the massage may only last for a few minutes if there is only a small area to be attended to or if time is pressing the participant to continue with competition. Ideally, the first inter-competition massage should be performed immediately after the first short cool-down. This massage should be fairly short – about 10 minutes. If required or desired, another short session can precede the next warm-up and so on throughout the competition. However, much more common is for the participant to appear midway through the day with a list of problems and the massage sessions must then be adapted to suit those needs and requirements.

Contraindications to Inter-Competition Massage

These are as previously stated in pre-competition massage. Be very vigilant and expect to find micro-trauma which must be referred to the appropriate professional.

Massage Post-Competition

At the end of training or competition the participant should perform the cool-down activity. Cool-down is the term used for the restoration of the body to its pre-exercise state. This should take place as soon after the cessation of the activity as possible. There are four distinct components to the cool-down:

1. Restore the cardiovascular system to its pre-activity level.
2. Rehydrate and refuel the body.
3. Remove the waste products from the muscle tissue.
4. Identify and treat any problems/injuries which have occurred.

Restore the cardiovascular system to its pre-activity level: This is accomplished by performing gradually diminishing exercise. A light jog, cycle or fairly brisk walk may suffice. However, if the participant is too exhausted to perform these activities or if injury precludes them, the medical team can provide a passive cool-down using passive movements and massage.

Rehydration and refuelling of the body: This is vitally important after strenuous activity and should be addressed as soon as possible. Fluid intake is of prime importance and the participant should be aware of the requirements. It may be only water or it may have to be some form of supplementation of minerals in a specialist drink or it may be a carbohydrate loaded drink.

Removal of waste products from the muscle tissue: This can be accomplished by gentle exercise and non-holding stretches, but be aware that the exercises to increase flexibility at the end of the activity may increase the stagnation of waste products in the tissues. If these are being performed they should be followed by gentle movements done in a rhythmical pattern.

Identify and treat injuries: Major injuries will be self-evident but minor problems and micro-tears are easily missed. The masseur is in an excellent position to address this problem, especially if the normal state of the participant's tissues is known. Any injury must be referred to the appropriate professional for accurate diagnosis before the masseur continues with their massage.

Objectives of Post-Competition Massage

To carry away waste products: As stated in inter-competition massage, the waste products can be successfully dispersed by massage. The main object is to influence circulation and increase the drainage action.

To help the body functions return to normal: After activity, the cardiovascular system may well be working very hard and the sudden cessation of activity can cause a drop in blood pressure. Massage, especially centripetal effleurage, can help to restore normality.

To prevent DOMS: Perform as previously described in Massage in Conditioning (*see* pages 81–4). Post-competition massage can be extremely useful in reducing and in some cases eliminating the post-activity muscle aches.

To work out 'niggles': Frequently after activity the participant may complain of certain specific areas of pain or tension. If any tissue damage or micro-tear has been diagnosed massage should only be administered after approval and discussion with the professional diagnostician. However, if the cause is purely exercise-induced, then massage is beneficial to remove the points of tightness.

Psychological Effect: At the end of competition the competitor will be either on a 'high' because the performance went well or, conversely, 'down' after a poor performance. The massage time can be used to give whichever help is called for, and as ever the importance of touch should not be underestimated.

Contact Materials to be Used in Post-Competition Massage

If it is possible the participant should have a shower prior to post-competition massage, although it may well be that this cannot be done because of lack of facility or the exhausted state of the participant. In the event of no shower having been taken the first action must be to clean the skin areas to be massaged. Again, for small areas wet tissues are ideal, but for whole limbs and large areas a spray bottle containing a mixture of water and liquid soap is best. Once the area has been cleansed, towel down gently and make use of the time to observe the skin condition. Massage lubricants used at this time will be light oils and/or creams. Those containing Arnica or, if available, non-steroidal anti-inflammatory agents are particularly good. If there is any fear of injury ice massage should be the application of choice. Do not use hot rubs or talcum powder as both are contraindicated. Hot rubs will exacerbate any micro-bleeds and talcum will slow down the cooling of the skin.

Techniques Used in Post-Competition Massage

This is the only time when massage can be used instead of active cool-down, and frequently has to replace activity by the participant. The most common times for this to occur are at the end of ultra-distance or endurance events, marathons, or if the participant is suffering from exhaustion. All manipulations must be applied slowly and rhythmically and to the depth that the participant finds tolerable.

Stroking GR1: This will accustom the participant to touch, and allow the masseur to assess

SPORTS MASSAGE APPLICATION

the skin condition, temperature, state of perspiration, and to identify any areas of tenderness or spasm.

- *Effleurage:* at first only GR1 and centripetal, then increased in depth and applied in all directions if there is no pain or tension and the participant is found to be at ease.

Petrissage: Kneading is the best of these manipulations to use and the depth should not exceed GR2. If there is no evidence of tender spots or spasms the other petrissage manipulations can be added one by one, but always pay attention to the participant's reaction and stop if there is any sign of pain or discomfort. The massage at this point is to reduce tension and help to return all the tissues to the pre-activity state.

Vibration: Performed to a maximum of GR2, vibration is very good, although again only if tolerated by the participant.

- *Effleurage:* This should be interspersed with the petrissage and applied for at least 5 minutes at the end of the session to enhance tissue drainage and give a good indication as to the final state of the tissues.

Remember that post-competition massage should never hurt.

Method of Application of Post-Competition Massage

Again, the purpose of massage will be to satisfy the requirements of the participant. Some may wish to have only one specific area, such as hamstrings, massaged. Others may want the whole body massaged and as previously stated the massage may have to replace the active cool-down period totally. This can often be a good time to reinforce advice on flexibility.

Duration of Post-Competition Massage

The time taken over post-competition massage very much depends on the area to be covered. If only a small part or one specific problem is to be addressed the time may be 15 to 30 minutes. For the whole body and when replacing the active cool-down the amount of time will vary – literally as long as it takes or as much time as is reasonably available. The results of this type of massage will be greatly enhanced by the use of a tepid shower or a not-too-hot jacuzzi. It is often advantageous to do part of the massage at the venue, return to base, have a shower and then have another short massage.

Contraindications to Post-Competition Massage

All previously listed contraindications apply. Be very circumspect around any painful areas, which may well be sites of trauma. Always seek advice and diagnosis as early as possible. If in doubt, use only ice-massage.

Massage Post-Travel

Sports people either in individual events or as members of a team will travel varying distances to participate in competition. In many cases their sport may take them all over the world. It is extremely difficult for a very active person to have to remain fairly static for any length of time and it is also easy to fret about training time that is being lost during travel. Whenever possible, sufficient time should be allowed to permit adequate acclimatization both to time changes and climatic conditions. A simple rule is one day for each hour of time alteration. In reality, however, the participants may not be able to allow for this time to acclimatize. The length of time spent on travel and the frequency of travel can therefore adversely affect performance. The major problems produced by travel in sport are:

- General feelings of stiffness.
- Feeling of lassitude.
- Aches, especially in the lower back, neck and shoulders.
- Swelling of lower legs and feet.

The solutions are:

- Light exercise
- Shower.
- Jacuzzi.
- Massage.

Objectives of Post-Travel Massage

To increase the venous and lymphatic flow: This will remove swelling and stiffness. Massage applied soon after the travel has been completed and especially after a gentle flexibility session, shower or jacuzzi can be very beneficial in the restoration of normal tissue state.

Gentle but deep massage to stretch the soft tissues: This will help to remove aches and increase flexibility.

To remove any residual stiffness: Massage can achieve this without tiring the participant through exercise or further stressing the cardiovascular system.

To restore the normal balance of the body: After a journey of any distance it is not unusual to feel restless and experience various aches, pains, cramps and 'odd sensations'. This is obviously more noticeable in the finely tuned athletic body and especially when the participant is

used to listening to the messages being received from muscle and soft tissue. Massage can relieve the various problems and speed up restoration to the norm.

To create a feeling of well-being: This is the usual psychological effect of massage and as stated before must not be underestimated.

Contact Materials to be Used in Post-Travel Massage

Fairly generous applications of oils and/or creams can be used at this time. Do not use hot rubs or talcum powders as there is still the possibility of the presence of dehydration and the necessity for the skin to get used to the temperature of the new environment.

Techniques Used in Post-Travel Massage

Stroking GR1 up to GR2: These are used to assess the condition of the skin, accustom the participant to touch and discover whether or not there is perspiration.

- *Effleurage:* Starting GR1 and deepening as tolerated. This is used at first only in the centripetal direction to aid tissue drainage and then progresses to multidirectional to promote tissue stretch.

Petrissage: Again, start light and then deepen to assist drainage and stretch the soft tissues. All techniques may be utilized.

- *Effleurage:* Use continually, regularly interspersed with all other strokes to reassess the tissue state and to assist drainage.

Tapotement, vibration and shaking: These may be applied all or individually to aid venous and lymphatic return and also to promote feelings of well-being.

- *Effleurage:* Use to end the session and reassess the final state of the tissues.

Method of Application of Post-Travel Massage

Start with the back and neck, then the legs and if necessary the arms as well. Spend more time on the trunk than usual as there can be a great deal of fluid stagnation in that area. If there is discernible lower limb swelling be sure to perform massage to the legs with the legs elevated so that drainage will be assisted. Encourage the participant to stretch gently at the end of the massage session.

Duration of Post-Travel Massage

This very much depends on the areas to be covered. If it is only legs 30 minutes will suffice, but if a whole body massage is to be administered the total time will be at least 1 hour. Should there be any swelling or drainage problems the massage should be administered until such time as there is a noticeable improvement of the condition. Better results from the massage will be gained if the participant has managed to have some gentle activity. A light, short jog, gentle swim, gentle stretches and then a tepid shower prior to the massage will give the best results.

Contraindications to Post-Travel Massage

All previously noted contraindications will apply. Pay particular attention to the state of hydration and be prepared to advise or seek help for this as necessary. If dealing with older participants or those with known circulation problems be on the look out for any venous problems, in particular deep venous thrombosis of the calf or lower limb, and if in any doubt, as always, get professional help to provide a diagnosis.

NON-SPECIFIC SPORTS MASSAGE

There are times when a participant will have no competition, conditioning has ceased and the sporting activities/training are nil or very much reduced. During all these times the athlete will still need to maintain the body in a state of preparedness for future conditioning and competition. Massage can play a very important part at this time and is referred to as non-specific sports massage.

This term may also apply to massage given when the participant has arrived at the competition site ahead of the event by at least 48 hours. The initial massage in the first 24 hours would be post-travel, but if massage was being used regularly thereafter for several days pre-competition it would be recorded as non-specific. Likewise, if the participant has completed all competition and is uninjured and appears for massage, this too is non-specific. Basically, we are referring to a massage which is given for no specific treatment purpose, and is not immediately before, between or after competition or travel. Non-specific sports massage can be divided into two applications:

1. General body massage.
2. Individual area/areas of massage.

General Body Massage

All people involved in sport at high or low levels are more aware of the actions and functions of muscle and joints. They spend a large part of their lives conditioning, preparing and training their bodies for the rigours of their particular sporting activity. Many of them are continually searching for that 'extra something' to give the edge to their performance. Massage is one aid that is very much appreciated and is often expected to deliver unrealistic effects. The use of regular massage throughout the participant's year, during training, conditioning and competition, has already been addressed. The use of massage during lay-off/rest periods is not well documented. Anecdotal evidence certainly seems to lead those involved both as masseurs and recipients to give a lot of credence to benefits gained from non-specific massage.

Objective of General Body Non-Specific Massage

To promote relaxation: If the participant's major request is to feel relaxed, then the massage should be administered with this aim in mind. Slow and rhythmical massage should be used to give the relaxation requested.

To provide stimulation: Again, if the participant feels that the body is sluggish because the normal level of activity is not taking place, the request may well be for a massage to provide stimulation. In this instance the main object is to produce an increase in circulation and muscle tone and the massage will be fast, deep and utilize all techniques to produce those effects.

To monitor the condition of the musculature and soft tissues: During a break in training the participant may become aware of areas that are 'not quite right'. This may well be increased muscle tone, connective tissue tension or long-standing fatigue. Massage, as well as highlighting these problems, can be effective in helping to reduce the symptoms.

To identify and then address any area where there is micro-scarring leading to reduced tissue flexibility: All sports people will suffer to a greater or lesser degree from tissue disruption because of the stress that the training schedule puts on the soft tissues. Non-specific massage can be utilized to ascertain the extent of these areas and help to produce the necessary stimulation of circulation and tissue mobility to increase flexibility.

The psychological effect: It is vital to ensure that the dedication and desire to succeed continues during any rest time. The contact with a knowledgeable masseur, especially one who knows and works regularly with the participant, can be invaluable. The feeling of something being achieved to improve the body state and enhance well-being is one of the main objectives of this type of massage.

Contact Materials to be Used in General Body Non-Specific Massage

The main criterion at this time is to go along with the preference of the participant, the only condition being that the lubricant must agree with the object of the massage. Oils, creams and powders, including the rubefacients, can be used. If the masseur is trained in aromatherapy the various preparations of essential oils will enhance the massage. Many participants still feel that the hotter the rub the better. This is not true and the masseur should take time to explain the adverse effects of too great a rise in superficial vaso-dilation.

Techniques Used in General Body Non-Specific Massage

Stroking GR1, followed by GR2 and then effleurage GR1: This will accustom the participant to touch and also assess the state of the tissues.

- *Effleurage:* If the massage is for relaxation it may be that the depth of these strokes does not increase above GR1 effleurage. Should relaxation not be achieved the depth may go to effleurage GR2. For relaxation the effleurage must be applied as

SPORTS MASSAGE APPLICATION

long, slow manipulations used continuously. In stimulative massage GR3, fast, shorter strokes are used.

Petrissage: This should start at GR1 and increase in depth to produce the desired effects. All the manipulations under this heading can be applied and the ones preferred by the participant should be used most.

Tapotement: Again this should be carried out to all levels and all manipulations as applicable to obtain the desired effects. Trigger pointing, acupressure and frictions can all be added. In some cases, the non-specific massage may have to change to a treatment massage if a specific problem is elicited.

- *Effleurage:* Whatever the object of the massage session the application must end with effleurage of reducing depth. This will ascertain the final tissue state and ensure there are no areas of tissue congestion remaining.

Method of Application of General Body Non-Specific Massage

Methods of application are as previously described in conditioning massage. The massage should begin with the back and neck, then each limb in turn and frequently foot massage. Some participants do not enjoy foot massage and in that case this should not be applied. The final stage of a general massage will be to return to the back and apply effleurage. If frictions, trigger pointing and acupressure are to be used, always apply effleurage to the area before finishing the massage.

Duration of General Body Non-Specific Massage

If the object of this massage is to produce relaxation the time taken will be dependent on that aim being achieved. This may well take between 1–1½ hours. It is important that the participant can lie and rest for at least half an hour after the completion of the massage. Never allow a participant to jump up immediately after a relaxing massage as they are liable to feel faint and/or dizzy. Stimulation will be achieved more quickly and the maximum for this type of massage is an hour. Dealing with problem areas will depend on the tolerance of the participant and may only take up a few moments of a whole massage.

Contraindictions to General Body Non-Specific Massage

All contraindications as previously listed will apply. Always obtain the proper professional help or diagnosis if there are any uncertainties or areas of problem identified.

Individual Area/Areas of Massage

Depending upon the muscle groups most used in their particular event, the participant may request an area of body to receive a massage, rather than a general body massage. For example, throwers and cricketers may wish to have their back and/or shoulders massaged, and any sports person who has to run may well feel the area to receive attention will be the hamstrings. Racquet players may wish calf and forearm muscles to be massaged. Whatever area requested must be addressed and the massage tailored to produce the desired effect.

Objectives of Individual Area Non-Specific Massage

These will be identical to general body non-specific massage. It is much more likely that a particular request to address an individual area will be targeted at a long-standing problem.

This would then require that area to be assessed and a diagnosis provided by the appropriate professional before sports massage could be started.

Contact Materials to be Used in Individual Area Non-Specific Massage

Again, this will very much depend on whether the massage is purely for relaxation or stimulation, or whether it changes into specific treatment. The full gambit of lubricants can apply if the massage is for relaxation or stimulation, but if altered to specific treatment these may be restricted as previously described.

Techniques Used in Individual Area Non-Specific Massage

The manipulations used will be as described in general body non-specific massage.

Method of Application of Individual Area Non-Specific Massage

The strokes applied will be in the same pattern as previously stated and applied only to the one area requested by the participant. Do ensure that the proximal areas are not congested. It is good practice to apply effleurage proximally before starting to deal with any specific area.

Duration of Individual Area Non-Specific Massage

This will be entirely dependent on achieving the desired results. The minimum time would be half an hour, but may need up to 1 hour on occasions.

Contraindications to Individual Area Non-Specific Massage

All contraindications as previously listed will apply. Be very sure to be in possession of an accurate diagnosis from the appropriate professional. The request for a individual area non-specific massage is almost certain to be aimed at an area that has been giving problems or to a known area of damage. Never start to massage unless you are sure you know what you are dealing with and that any injury or long-standing problem area has been accurately identified by the appropriate professional. Never give a first massage to a participant within 48 hours of competition, and always arrange for the first-ever massage to take place when there is plenty of time (72+ hours) for any adverse effects to be worked off. These adverse effects may be: producing too much relaxation, stirring up old problems such as scar tissue, or reactions to the lubricants used.

Sports massage is generally sport-specific and any masseur involved must know and understand the principles of that sport. Most importantly, the rules, regulations and call-up times of the sport must be understood.

There will not always be time to perform the beginning, middle and end of a massage in the sharp-end situation. The masseur must be prepared to give as good a massage as possible with the proviso of producing the result required and adhering to the rules as much as possible.

The most important issue in a situation where time is limited is to be absolutely clear about the main object of that massage. It may be to eliminate a particular point of tension or to increase range of movement. Once this object has been identified, select which of the techniques can best deliver the desired effect and use them. Remember, if the sport is taking place outdoors, for example orienteering, skiing or rugby, it may not even be possible to remove clothing. In such instances, whole-limb shaking, vibrations and trigger pointing through the clothing will be the best manipulations to use.

CHAPTER 6
Additional Massage Techniques

More and more masseurs are adding to their skills by using additional techniques.

ADDITIONAL MASSAGE TECHNIQUES

The three most common additions are:
1. Ice massage.
2. Aromatherapy massage
3. Reflexology.

Ice Massage

As the name implies, the massage in this instance is applied with the use of ice. The ice used may be just a cube of ice, it may be a container holding a block of ice, or it may be a polythene bag filled with crushed ice.

Objective of Ice Massage

To promote recovery from micro-trauma: As previously stated, it is common to sustain small tears when training or competing in sport at any level. The use of ice massage when any such trauma is suspected or has been diagnosed is very helpful.

To cool the participant down: The participant may have experienced overheating through sustained effort or because the training/competition has taken place in high temperature or humidity. In these instances, the great risk

is heat exhaustion. Application of ice packs either round the body or as a massage can be employed with excellent results.

Before friction massage: Providing there has been an accurate diagnosis obtained and friction is recommended, ice massage will numb the tissue prior to the friction. This is particularly useful if the participant finds the area to be frictioned too tender to tolerate the friction.

After friction massage: The object of transverse friction may well be to break down adherent scar tissue. At first, the friction will produce a numbing effect. When the frictions cease there may be mild bleeding in the tissue and the participant may experience pain. Ice massage will help slow/stop the bleeding and continue the numbing sensation.

Contact Materials to be Used in Ice Massage

When using an ice cube to apply ice massage, the area to be massaged should first be cleaned, and a little oil applied to the skin. Likewise with a container of ice and a bag of ice the application of a small amount of oil will facilitate the movement and protect the skin.

A very useful container for ice massage application is a polystyrene cup. This is filled with water, allowed to freeze and then when needed a small strip about 2cm deep is cut from the top rim. The ice stands proud and

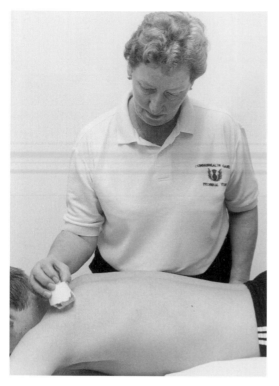

Fig 120. Polystyrene cup to apply ice massage.

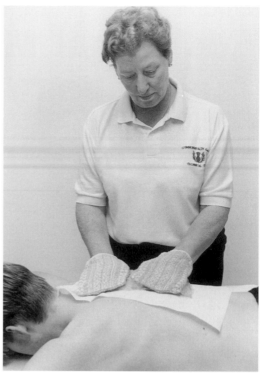

Fig 121. Towelling mittens to protect hands.

the masseur can hold the rest of the cup in his or her hand (Fig 120). When using a cube or polythene bag a towelling mitten is needed to protect the masseur's hand (Fig 121).

Techniques Used in Ice Massage and Method of Application

Stroking: Ice massage should always start proximal to the suspected area of damage. Use only two to four centripetal strokes and then do the same distally. Follow with light strokes over the area.

Kneading: Circular kneading-type movements can be applied over and around the area if this can be tolerated.

Stroking: To end the session stroke the ice from distal to proximal, that is, centripetal. If dealing with a limb have the limb in an elevated position throughout the massage.

Duration of Ice Massage

Duration should be only for a few minutes, and always stop if there is any sign of skin reddening or irritation. It is best if the participant can report that the area is numb, but sometimes the skin reaction will prevent this occurring.

Contraindications of Ice Massage

All previous contraindications should be remembered, but on this occasion the massage will most often be applied as the direct result of injury.

Remember that an accurate diagnosis must first have been established by the appropriate professional. Any history of circulatory problem should immediately be referred to that professional.

Aromatherapy Massage

Aromatherapy is the therapeutic use of substances bearing odours which are obtained from plants, flowers and fragrant shrubs. These substances are generally referred to as essential oils. The extraction and preparation of these oils is not within the scope of this publication and only those therapists trained and skilled should attempt to engage in this activity. There are many different oils available and only the purest should be used and obtained from reputable sources. Essential oils can be administered in several different ways. They may be added to a warm bath, inhaled as a vapour, taken internally or massaged into the skin.

In sports massage a limited number of essential oils can be safely used by the masseur for therapeutic reasons or to give a more pleasant smell to the lubricant. The oils to be used are dissolved in a carrier oil and used as the massage lubricant. Just how much essential oil will penetrate the skin is still the subject of debate and research. The absorption of oils will vary with the various skin types encountered. A suggested dilution is three to twelve drops of essential oil to 30ml of carrier oil. If the oil has dilution quantities on the label always follow this advice. Vegetable oil is a good base carrier oil.

Objectives of Aromatherapy Massage in Sport

Relaxation: The best and main use of this par-

ticular form of massage in sport is to help provide relaxation.

To aid nasal congestion: Frequently sports people complain of nasal congestion, especially if competing indoors. In these circumstances a few drops of peppermint or eucalyptus oil added at the end of a massage can help to reduce the problem.

Stress relief: This is one of the main objects addressed by the usage of essential oils.

Stimulation and invigoration: These can be aided by the use of rosemary and lemon oils.

Psychological effects: As previously stated, these must not be underestimated in any massage. The addition of a pleasant odour to the massage can only enhance the general feeling of well-being produced by the massage.

Contact Materials to be Used in Aromatherapy Massage

The carrier oil must first be chosen. There are several from which to select, depending on the properties required. The most frequently used are listed below.

Almond oil: A light, fairly reasonably priced, easily obtainable oil which keeps well. It is soothing and softening, and can be used on the body and face.

Avocado oil: A heavy, expensive oil, obtainable at specialist outlets, best bought in small quantities as it breaks down readily. It is deeply penetrating and nourishing, good for dry and mature skin. Use on the body and sparingly on the face.

Corn oil: A medium to heavy oil, reasonably priced and easily obtainable. It keeps fairly well, and is nourishing to use on the body.

Grapeseed oil: A fine, very reasonably priced oil which is easily obtainable and keeps well. This oil has no smell, which can be an advantage. It is nourishing and can be used on both the body and face.

Jojoba oil: A medium to heavy, slightly more expensive but easily obtainable oil which keeps well. It is very nourishing, and is good for dry and mature skins. Use on the body and face.

Olive oil: A very heavy oil, expensive but easily obtainable and keeps well. It is nourishing and can be used on the body.

Peach/apricot kernel oil: Both have similar properties. They are fairly heavy oils, very expensive, and only obtainable at specialist outlets. They keep well. Use these deeply penetrating oils on the face.

Sunflower oil: A light, inexpensive, easily obtainable oil which keeps well. It is nourishing and can be used on both the body and face.

Wheatgerm oil: A heavy, sticky oil which prevents other oils from going rancid as it contains vitamin E. It is slightly more expensive but easily obtainable and keeps well. A nourishing oil, use on both the body and face.

Essential oils most used in sports massage are:

Basil: Used for pain relief, basil eases muscle spasm and is regarded as a refreshing oil.

Benzoin: Used for pain relief, benzoin reduces inflammation, stimulates circulation, and is regarded as a relaxing oil.

Bergamot: Used for pain relief, bergamot eases muscle spasm, and is regarded as both a refreshing and relaxing oil.

Cajeput: Used for pain relief, cajeput eases muscle spasm, and is regarded as a warming oil.

Camphor: Used for pain relief, camphor eases muscle spasm, stimulates circulation, and is regarded as a stimulating oil.

Chamomile: Used for pain relief, especially muscular aches and pains, chamomile reduces inflammation, and is regarded as both a refreshing and relaxing oil.

Eucalyptus: Used for pain relief, especially muscular, eucalyptus eases muscle spasm, purifies the blood of toxins and waste products, stimulates circulation, clears the head, and is regarded as a refreshing oil.

Geranium: Used for pain relief, geranium eases muscle spasm, reduces inflammation, and is regarded as both a refreshing and relaxing oil.

Lavender: Used for pain relief, lavender eases muscle spasm, reduces inflammation, and is regarded as both a refreshing and relaxing oil.

Lemon: Used for pain relief, lemon stimulates circulation, and is regarded as a stimulating oil.

Marjoram: Used for pain relief, especially muscular aches and pain, marjoram reduces muscle spasm, and is regarded as a warming oil.

Peppermint: Used for pain relief, peppermint reduces inflammation, clears the nose, and is regarded as a refreshing oil.

Rosemary: Used for pain relief, rosemary

stimulates the circulation, and is regarded as both a refreshing and stimulating oil.

Sandalwood: Used to ease muscle spasm and reduce inflammation, sandalwood is regarded as a relaxing oil.

There are many more essential oils, but the above list tends to cover those most frequently used by the sports masseur.

Techniques Used in Aromatherapy Massage in Sport

All of the techniques previously described under the stroking manipulations and petrissage manipulations can be used. Frictions, tapotement and shaking are not applied. Acupressure and trigger pointing can also be used as part of aromatherapy sports massage.

Method of Application of Aromatherapy Massage in Sport

This will depend on the objective of the massage. Most often, this type of massage will be used at the end of the conditioning phase or as a non-specific general body massage. The methods will be as previously described.

Duration of Aromatherapy Massage in Sport

In most cases when aromatherapy is used in sport, it will be as a full body massage. The time spent is therefore going to be at least 1 hour. If the oils are being added at the end of another type of massage it may be that the aromatherapy part of the massage actually only lasts for a few moments.

Contraindications to Aromatherapy Massage in Sport

All the contraindications to massage previ-

ously listed will apply. It is also wise to be aware of the possibility of allergic reactions. Be very careful that essential oils do not come into contact with the eyes. If oil does get into the eyes, it should be washed out with distilled water and medical help sought.

Some oils do have their own contraindications. Of the essential oils listed, bergamot can produce photosensitivity, so should not be used when the participant is going to be training or competing in the sunshine. Chamomile can give a slight chance of producing dermatitis. Geranium also has a slight risk of producing sensitivity. Rosemary should be avoided during pregnancy and if epileptic. Generally, anyone who has an allergic reaction to perfume is likely to be allergic to essential oils. If participants suffer from skin or other allergies always check with the doctor and a qualified aromatherapist before using any essential oils. **Do not use cheap oils and always obtain further advice if there are any doubts**.

The use of essential oils in sports massage is to enhance the effect of the massage. In no way should the masseur use the oils in the same manner as a properly trained aromatherapist unless he or she has been trained in the full usage of these oils.

Reflexology

This is a system of diagnosis and treatment which originates in China and India. Like most of the Eastern methods it dates back thousands of years. Reflexology is based on the belief that the whole body is represented on the soles of the feet. These reflexology zones on the feet do not correspond exactly to the nervous system (Fig7 122). As in traditional Chinese medicine, the principle of illness due to energy channel blockage applies. Reflexology is believed to encourage natural healing of the mind and body, by pressure and deep massage.

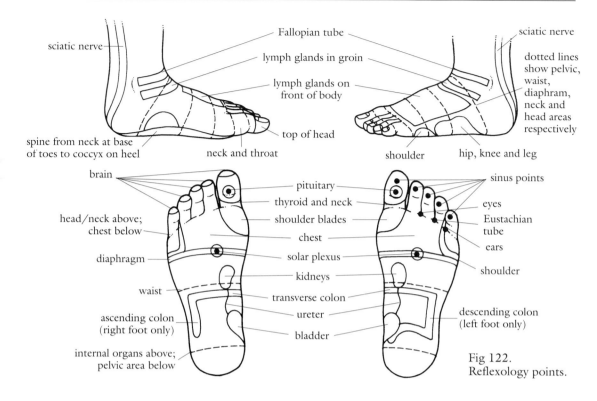

Fig 122.
Reflexology points.

Objectives of Reflexology in Sports Massage

Relaxation: The main purpose of the use of reflexology in sports massage is to provide relaxation.

Identifying problem areas: Any problem area will be identified by some feeling of discomfort when the appropriate reflex point is palpated.

Tension relief: Reflexology can be extremely effective in providing relief for back, neck and general tension problems.

Psychological effect: As stated before, many participants enjoy a general foot massage at the end of a massage session. Some will find greater benefits from the use of reflexology techniques.

Contact Material Used in Reflexology

The only lubricant to be used in reflexology should be a little talcum powder.

Techniques Used in Reflexology

As in many branches of complementary massage, the terminology used to describe the massage manipulations is different from that already described. There are eight different types of massage manipulation commonly used in reflexology:

1. The caterpillar movement.
2. The rotation action.
3. The stroking or milking movement.
4. The feather or healing movement.
5. Scrunching.
6. Spinal scrunch or twist.

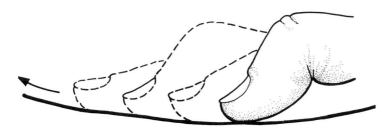

Fig 123. Caterpillar movement.

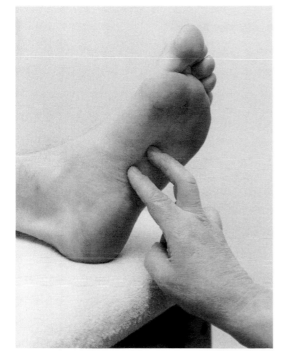

Fig 124. Caterpillar movement being applied.

7. Toe rotating.
8. Circular caress.

The caterpillar movement: This is performed by the tips and pads of the thumbs and fingers (Fig 123). Contact is made with the tips of both thumbs and fingers, and then the pads rest lightly on the skin. The hand is then rocked forwards so that the pad loses contact and the tip only touches. Without breaking contact, move the thumb or finger forward and repeat the action from tip to pad and back to tip. Also called thumb walking (Fig 124).

The rotation action: This is a finger or thumb kneading action performed on the reflex points (Fig 125). The thumb tips or finger tips are placed on the reflex points and vibrated without moving the digits. Light pressure can be used on the reflex point and held for a few seconds. As the pressure is released the fingers and thumb rotate (Fig 126).

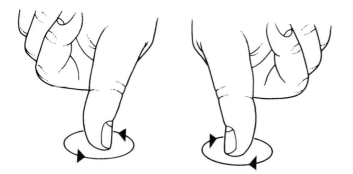

Fig 125. Rotation movement.

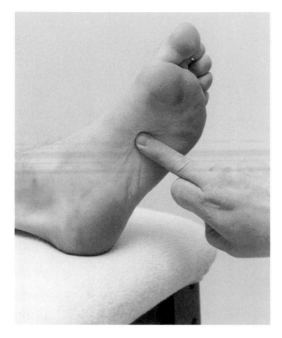

Fig 126. Rotation movement being applied.

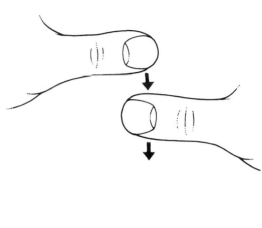

Fig 127. Stroking or milking movement.

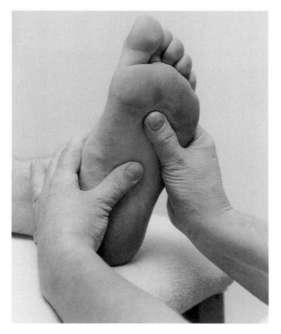

Fig 128. Stroking or milking movement being applied.

The stroking or milking movement: Again, the fingers or thumbs are used to stroke the reflex points (Fig 127). The strokes can be long or short and slight pressure is applied (Fig 128). This movement may be performed using the whole hand. One hand cups the sole of the foot and the other is placed on top of the foot (Fig 129). Slowly stroke from toes to ankle and down again (Fig 131).

The feather or healing movement: This is also a stroking manipulation, very similar to the thousand hands technique (Fig 130). To be applied very lightly.

Scrunching: Hold the foot firmly between the fingers and thumb of each hand. Start just under the toes and twist each hand in opposite directions. Work from the toes to the ankle (Fig 132).

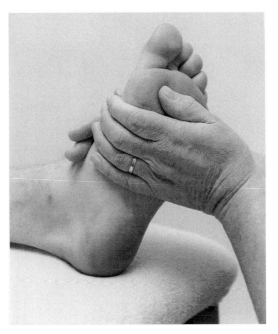

Fig 129. Stroking or milking movement using the whole hand.

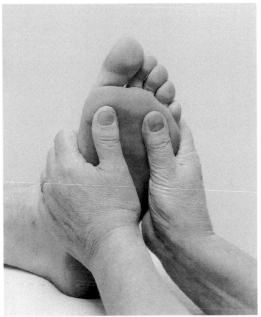

Fig 130. Feather or healing movement being applied.

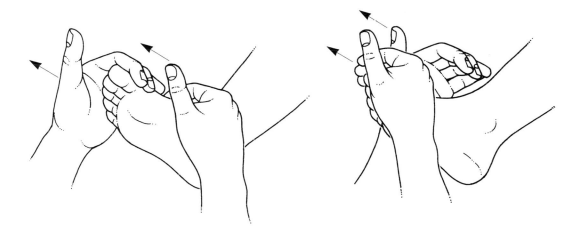

Fig 131. Stroking or milking movement – direction.

Spinal scrunch or twist: Both hands rest on the top of the foot with thumbs touching on the sole (Fig 133). The hand nearest to the toes is moved backwards and forwards to twist gently the spinal reflex.

Toe rotating: One thumb is placed on the diaphragm point at the base of the toe level. The other hand is used to gently rotate the toes (Fig 134).

Circular caress: The heel of the hand or the fist may be used to perform this manipulation (Figs 135 & 136). Press the heel of the hand into the ball of the foot and slowly rotate, or make a fist and press the back of the fingers into the ball of the foot and slowly rotate.

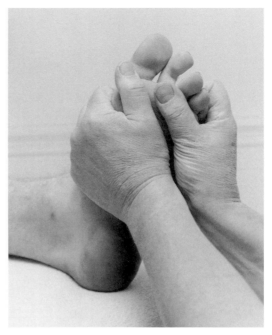

Fig 132. Scrunching.

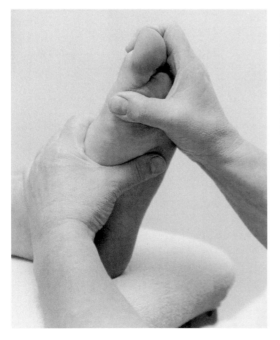

Fig 133. Spinal scrunch or twist.

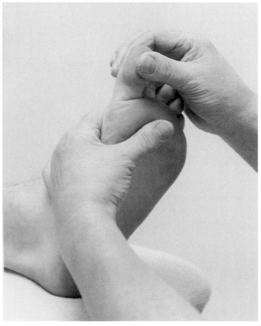

Fig 134. Toe rotating.

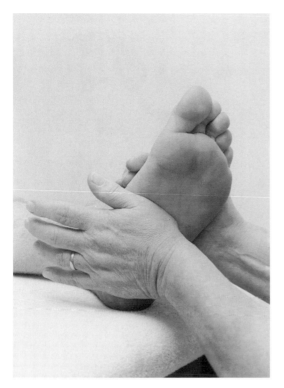

Fig 135. Circular caress using heel of hand.

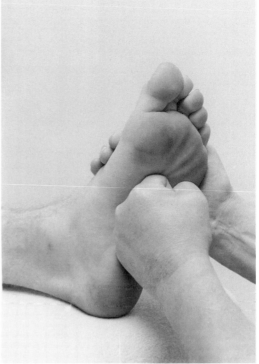

Fig 136. Circular caress using fist.

*Method of Application of Reflexology
in Sports Massage*

Both feet should be massaged, and most benefit is gained by starting with the dominant side and then the other foot and returning to the dominant again if needed. The stroking or milking movement should always start the massage. The caterpillar or thumb walk is applied next. The feather or healing movement is best used interspersed between other movements.

Scrunching, spinal scrunch or twist, rotation action, toe rotating and circular caress may all be used, or only some as judged necessary. Pay attention to which manipulation the participant finds irritating or painful and be prepared to stop if real discomfort is experienced. The stroking or milking movement should be used at the end of the massage session.

Duration of Reflexology in Sports Massage

The true reflexologist who uses this method of complementary healing to influence mind, body and soul will spend up to 2 hours on one session. In the world of sports massage, reflexology is used as part of the battery of skills to give relaxation and as such a much shorter time is spent performing it. Quite often at the end of a particularly hard training day or conditioning session just 10 minutes of this massage will give excellent results.

*Contraindications to Reflexology
in Sports Massage*

All of the well-trained reflexologists agree that it is impossible to cause harm with reflexology. It is good practice, however, to remember all the previously listed contraindications to massage. In particular, when dealing with sports people it is very common to find feet that suffer from fungal infections. This should be a total contraindication to reflexology because of the risk of spread of infection. It is also not unusual to find blisters and/or burst blisters. These areas would be too painful to massage and also give the risk of introducing infection.

The major warnings given about reflexology are that palpitations, hyperventilation or panic may be aroused from the subconscious effect of the treatment. The response is to calm the person and encourage relaxation. At the end of the massage the participant should be encouraged to drink water to flush out any extra toxins. This also ties in well with the rehydration of the sports participant.

There are very many alternative methods of massage available, but ice massage, aromatherapy and reflexology are the ones most associated with sports massage. Ice massage is quite easy to explain and can be applied by most people with only a scant knowledge and observation of very obvious precautions. Aromatherapy, on the other hand, is a science in its own right. If the essential oils are to be used in all their applications and prepared by the masseur, then that masseur must be trained to the recognized standard by the appropriate authority. The small part in this chapter is to allow the masseur to try to use already prepared oils to enhance the massage used, but is not intended to make the reader a qualified aromatherapist.

Reflexology is also one of the many Eastern forms of medicine. Like aromatherapy, it is also worthy of full study. The snippet described here is again to give an alternative to the sports masseur but does not provide the extensive training undertaken by the qualified reflexologist.

CHAPTER 7
Other Massage Modalities

To the purist in massage there is only one method of applying massage and that is by hand. However, in the world of sport there is a very large and thriving market introducing many new and innovative 'massage modalities'. The serious sports masseur will find that there are some modalities which, although they will never replace the 'hands on' massage, can be beneficial to the participant.

OTHER MASSAGE MODALITIES

These can best be dealt with under three headings:

1. Electrically powered massagers.
2. Water-based massage.
3. Massage applicators.

Electrically Powered Massagers

These can come in a wide range of shapes, sizes and cost, from the tiny battery-operated vibrating massager up to the large, free-standing saloon model. There are two different types of electrically operated massagers.

Percussors

These function on a vertical plane and produce an up and down movement which can best be compared to that obtained by using tapotement. They come in all sizes from small, hand-held applicators to massage belts, vibrating cushions and chairs. Although popular among many sports people, they really do not produce such good effects as gyrators in the area of sports massage (Fig 137).

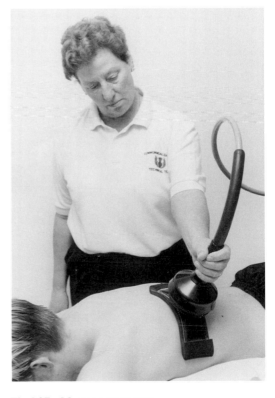

Fig 137. Massage percussor.

Gyrators

These function on a horizontal plane and most closely resemble the massage action of the human hand. The action of this electrical massager produces a movement which simulates effleurage if used in a stroking motion, and petrissage if applied in a circular pattern.

This type of massager is widely used in North America both in sports clinics and hospitals. In Great Britain, these massagers traditionally are still more popular in the beauty therapy world. There has, however, in the last two to three years been an upsurge in their usage in sport in this country. Many well-renowned soccer teams now include both the large stand model and hand-held portable model in their sports clinics (Figs 138 & 139).

Unlike the percussors, the gyrators can be used with good effect in sports massage. The main advantage over hand massage is two-fold – time-saving and requiring less energy output from the masseur. Both of these may be very valid advantages if time is limited and there is only one masseur to massage a large team.

Most participants will readily accept an electrically operated massager if that is all that is on offer. The small hand-held unit can also be self-administered by the participant, provided they can adopt a comfortable non-stressed position to apply the massage. This, in turn, can make these items useful to the

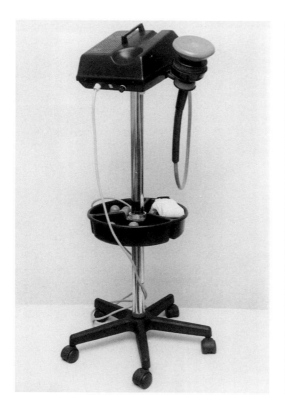

Fig 138. Stand model gyrator massager.

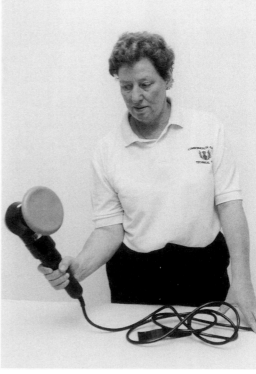

Fig 139. Hand-held gyrator massager.

participant who travels alone and has no access to a sports masseur. A complete body massage with a gyrator will only take about 20 minutes as opposed to the 1–1½ hours required for traditional massage.

Objectives of Electrically Produced Massage in Sport

Maintaining mobility in soft tissue: The type of tissue movement produced by massagers will maintain mobility in the soft tissue structures. This is very useful for mobilizing scar tissue, and can also prepare for warm-up.

To increase blood flow: The higher frequency vibration will cause vasodilatation of the blood vessels and result in increased blood flow. It can also aid cool-down.

Muscle relaxation: The rhythmical action is effective in producing muscle relaxation. It can also be used during travel and cool-down.

Trigger points: Trigger points can be successfully stimulated by the application of a single pointer applicator.

Psychological effect: The sensations produced by the massagers are usually pleasantly acceptable and therefore do produce some psychological effects. This is not nearly so obvious as the result of hand-applied massage and frequently the two types of massage used successively will produce the better result.

Contact Materials to be Used with Electrical Massagers

Previously, manufacturers recommended that only a very small amount of talcum powder should be used with massagers. Now applicator covers, both disposable and reusable, are available. This enables the use of oils, lotions and creams with the massager. Specially prepared 'sports massage' lotions and creams are often recommended by the manufacturers. Only use them if you are happy with their content. The usual oil or lotion used by the masseur can be applied with the electrical massager. Do not use as much as you would in hand-applied massage and avoid very fine or very heavy oils. Always use the applicator cover if using any lubricant.

Techniques Used with Electrical Massagers in Sports Massage

Most electrical massagers will be supplied with instructions, detailing the particular usage of each machine. The techniques used to best effect in sport are a slow stroking-type movement and circular kneading-type movement. Trigger pointing can be applied very well with the correct applicator (Fig 140).

Method of Application of Electrical Massager in Sport

It is essential always to follow the manufacturer's instructions. The correct applicator should be selected and the protective cover applied. Initial contact is best made with a U-shaped applicator or the applicator provided for general usage (Figs 141 & 142). The massager should be held in one hand and the other hand used to palpate the tissue ahead of the applicator (Fig 143). If the participant is thin a towel is best applied over the area to be massaged or the applicator cover can be used (Fig 144). The applicator should be held in one area and then moved to the adjoining area with a slight lift between. Never press hard or try to manipulate the applicator.

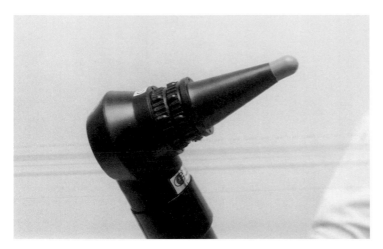

Fig 140. Applicator for trigger pointing.

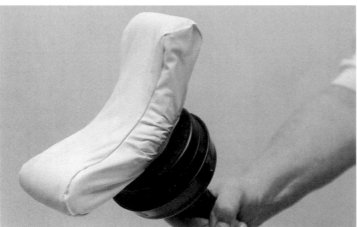

Fig 141. U-shaped applicator.

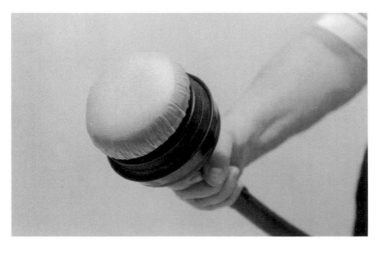

Fig 142. General applicator.

Fig 143. Massager in use with hand palpating ahead.

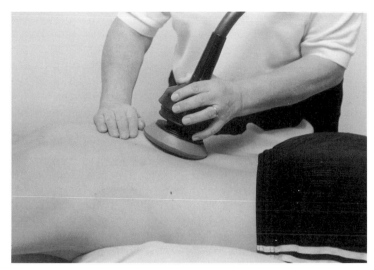

Fig 144. Cover over applicator head.

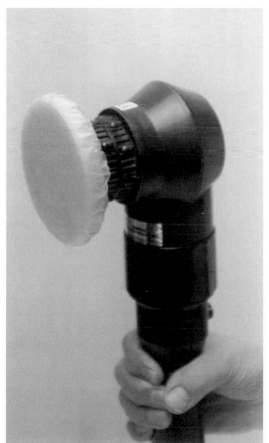

Always work from distal to proximal. When addressing very muscular legs or back use a two- or four-ball applicator or multipronged applicator (Figs 145, 146 & 147). For trigger pointing use the conical or narrowest applicator set to about 40 to 50 cycles per second. Hold the point between the first two fingers of your hand (Fig 148). Apply the point for 10 to 15 seconds and then release, continue to apply to the one point for a maximum of 2 minutes and then move on to another point, returning to the first later if it is still active. Finish the application with a general stroking with either a U-shape or large soft circular applicator.

Duration of Electrical Massage in Sport

As previously stated, a complete body massage will take 20 to 30 minutes, while trigger pointing will depend on the release of the active trigger point. I have found that the best results are obtained by 10 to 15 seconds application, interspersed with 5 to 10 second rests, repeated for a maximum of 2 minutes.

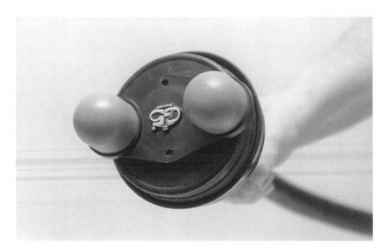

Fig 145. Two-ball applicator.

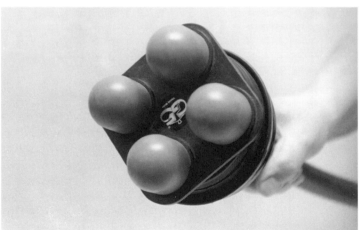

Fig 146. Four-ball applicator.

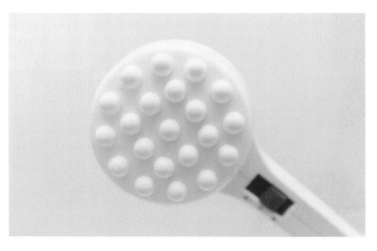

Fig 147. Multipronged applicator.

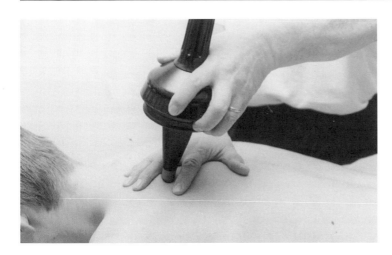

Fig 148. Trigger pointer being applied.

If necessary, move to another point and then reapply once more in the same sequence.

If the participant is to apply the massager to themselves, I instruct an application of general usage of 15 minutes. For specific points, I recommend two sets of 2 minutes duration in 15 second bursts with a rest of 2 minutes between each set.

Contraindications to Electrical Massagers

All contraindications as previously listed apply. Safety procedures applicable to electrical apparatus must be observed. In particular, all machines must be regularly serviced and maintained according to the manufacturers instructions. All legal safety obligations must be met. Never use the massager in the shower or bath. Most small machines are best used only for 15 to 20 minutes at a time and should not be allowed to overheat. Make sure the applicators and covers are cleaned before each application. If there is any possible risk of soft tissue injury be sure to get the proper diagnosis and consent to apply the massage before commencing.

Water-Based Massage

Like hand-applied massage, the use of water or baths to aid preparation for and recovery from exercise can be traced back to Roman times. Steam baths were also used in Turkey, whilst in Scandinavian countries the sauna was used. Originally the 'spa' bath was used to cleanse the body and provide relaxation. In Far Eastern countries, Japan in particular, hot baths were part of the social scene as well as being used therapeutically.

Many modern sports complexes and hotels provide saunas, Turkish baths, various jacuzzis and spa baths. These can be utilized by the sports masseur to aid the effects of massage, or in the instances when the participant does not have access to a masseur they may be instructed in the usage of 'baths' to at least give some help.

Techniques Used in Water/Steam-Based Massage

Sauna: Use of a sauna post-competition or post-conditioning can be beneficial to help clear waste products. The use of cold plunge pools or massage with snow as used in Scandinavia after a sauna will cause superficial vessels to vasoconstrict and can elevate blood pressure. Saunas can also be used to aid acclimatization if going to train or compete in a humid climate.

Turkish baths/other steam baths: The most common usage of steam baths in sport is to assist participants in 'making weight' in weight category sports, for example loss of weight for boxers, weight-lifters and so on who must not be above a certain weight level for competition. This is not to be recommended and all in all the effects of such activity can be extremely debilitating. Any usage in sport should be at the participant's instigation and not during the active phase of competition. These steam baths can also be utilized as part of acclimatization training.

Spa bath/jacuzzi: These may be a normal domestic bath with a special perforated base. This is connected to an electrically operated air compressor. The bath is filled, the compressor is activated and warm air is forced through the holes in the base of the bath. This can be very relaxing, help to reduce muscle spasms, open up pores and cleanse waste products. The commercial-style jacuzzi found in hotel and leisure complexes is just a larger version of the one described here.

The next most common spa bath is the aerated bath. This is usually an individual deep bath which is filled with warm water. To this may be added any aromatherapy oil, remembering which effect each specific oil can give, either relaxation or stimulation. In some spas seaweed is used, or where there are natural mineral or thermal springs, that water will be utilized. The whole bath is then aerated with oxygen from a compressor unit which forms part of the spa bath. The participant lies in this bath for a maximum of 15

minutes whilst their body is bombarded by little bubbles.

Some spas will have a selection of 'shower cabinets' which can deliver various types of water spray. This may simply consist of a high-pressure shower-head with a facility to alter the outlet from a normal watering-can-type spray to one or several pulsating outlets. More sophisticated shower cabinets will have jets of water coming from the roof and/or walls of the cabinet. There is usually the facility to choose which jets one wishes to have on. The major advantage of this type of spa shower in sport is that it can be used during competition or training without resulting in the lethargy which often follows the use of saunas and jacuzzis.

Method of Application of Water/Steam-Based Massage

Sauna: Only use when training/competition has been completed and always follow the manufacturer's instructions. Allow plenty of time so that it is possible to have a shower and rest for up to 30 minutes after the sauna.

Turkish/steam baths: Do not use prior to competition or hard training. These can be most effective once or twice a week after an easy training session. Again, allow time to shower and rest as above.

Spa bath/jacuzzi: These are particularly useful after travel, heavy training and post-competition. Prior to non-specific or general body massage these baths can enhance the effects of hand-applied massage. It is always good practice to shower after the bath and prior to any hand-on massage.

Aerated baths: These are also most efficacious prior to general body massage. They can produce a feeling of lethargy or relaxation. They are best used after travel, and post-competition and training.

Shower units: These are either general shower units or can be used to stimulate specific areas. Providing hydration is maintained and the water is not too warm they can be used prior to pre-competition massage and warm-up. They are also very good for post-competition cool-down.

Duration of Water/Steam-Based Massage

Sauna: Always obey the manufacturer's instructions. The advice to sports participants is to limit sauna usage time to a maximum of 15 minutes at the lowest comfortable temperature and only 5 minutes at their own maximum tolerance.

Turkish/steam baths: The majority of commercially used units are connected to time-control units to prevent overexposure. First-time usage should be limited to 10 minutes, rising to a maximum of 25 minutes as acclimatization is reached.

Spa bath or jacuzzi: The maximum usage should be 15 minutes. The higher the water temperature, the shorter the exposure time must be.

Aerated baths: Again, most units are connected to time-mechanisms to prevent overuse. The average recommended time would be 10 to 15 minutes. Again, the higher the water temperature, the shorter the exposure time. The type of oils used may also affect the duration.

Shower units: If using a specific pin-point shower the time must be limited by the participant's own reaction – for example when the point feels numb or relaxed cease usage of the shower. A generalized spray or jet should not exceed 10 minutes.

Contraindications to Water/Steam Massage in Sport

All previously listed contraindications apply. Select the modality to be used with great care to enhance performance. Sauna, Turkish, steam, spa, jacuzzi or aerated baths should not be used before or during competition. Never start any water or steam-based massage for the first time within 72 hours of competition or training. Always observe all of the manufacturer's rules and health and safety regulations as are applicable. Remember to rest and relax for up to 30 minutes after a sauna, Turkish, steam, aerated bath or jacuzzi, then have a shower. This is essential to permit any excess perspiring to stop and allow the heart rate to return back to normal.

Massage Applicators

Applicators for massage are produced in a plethora of guises. They are made from wood, plastic, sponge, bristles and cloth such as towelling. The majority of such applicators tend to be gimmicky fashion items with no part to play in the life of the serious masseur. There are, however, some applicators which can be used to help the sport participant and, in particular, the participant who wants to or has to apply self-massage.

Many experts and books on sports massage recommend self-administered massage. However, it is extremely difficult to apply self-massage. Firstly, it is difficult to be able to relax the area to be massaged whilst applying the massage to oneself. Secondly, many body areas cannot be reached even by the most accomplished contortionist. However, when a sports participant requires a massage and no masseur is available then self-massage may be the only option. In such instances some applicators may help to give a more acceptable massage and produce better results than hands-on.

A long-handled applicator (Fig 149) can be used to reach the backs of the legs and the backs of the shoulders without placing undue

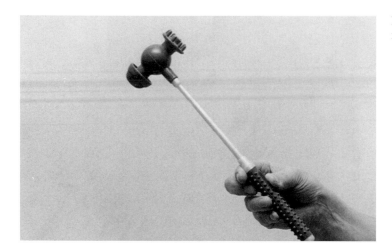

Fig 149. Long-handled massage applicator.

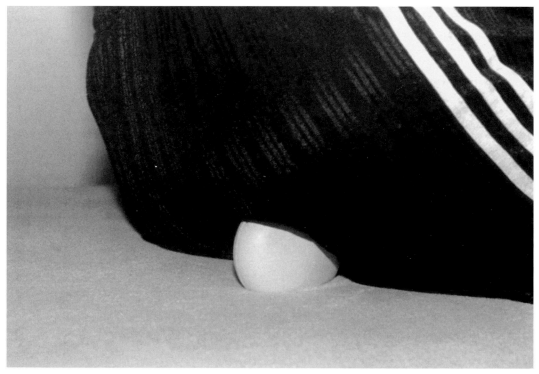

Fig 150. Buttock trigger pointing with ball.

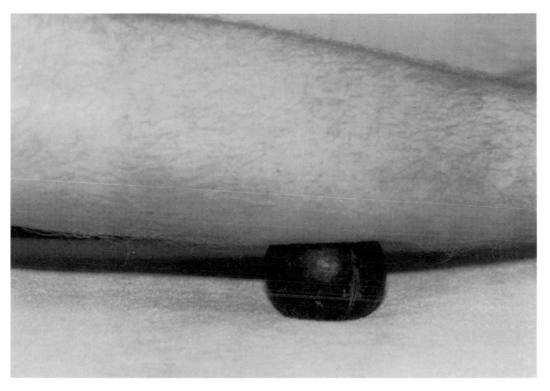

Fig 151. Calf trigger pointing with ball.

stresses on other parts of the body. A ladder-like arrangement of wooden balls can be used very effectively to administer massage to the upper shoulders, thorax and lumbar areas.

Perhaps the most advantageous applicators are round. A tennis ball, a wooden ball, a squash ball and even a large inflatable exercise ball can be used to good effect. A ball can be positioned under or over a trigger point and pressure applied. For trigger points in the buttock area the participant can sit on the ball

and apply pressure (Fig 150). Under a tight calf (Fig 151) it works very well, and also on the upper shoulders when applied with the other hand. As the pressure is self-administered the risk of injury is remote.

The remit of the sports masseur in self-massage either with or without an applicator is to ensure that the participant is aware of the contraindications to all massage and that they do not cause themselves any harm or injury from overzealous application.

CHAPTER 8
Anatomy and Physiology Revision

As stated in Chapter 2, it is not the purpose of this book to provide the in-depth knowledge needed to understand anatomy and physiology, or to give diagnostic skills. The sports masseur should, however, have a very good working knowledge of practical anatomy and a basic understanding of physiology.

The intention of this final chapter is to provide a ready reference to support prior learning. The sports masseur must never be afraid to check up exactly which structure or muscle is giving problems, especially if access to a competent diagnostician is not readily available. Far safer and more effective massage will be applied if the sports masseur is competent in identifying the surface anatomy and is aware of the basic actions of that particular body part.

Anatomy: Anatomy deals with the structure of the body and the relationship of the various components to each other.

Physiology: Physiology deals with the study of the body parts. For the purposes of this book and to allow easy reference the body is divided into five major and four minor systems.

Major systems:
1. Skeletal system.
2. Muscular system.
3. Vascular system.
4. Lymphatic system.
5. Neurological system.

Minor systems:
1. Digestive system.
2. Respiratory system.
3. Genito-urinary system.
4. Endocrine system.

MAJOR SYSTEMS – SKELETAL SYSTEM

The adult skeleton consists of 206 bones (Figs 152 & 153). There are five different types of bone:

1. Long bones such as the femur in the thigh, and humerus in the upper arm.
2. Short bones such as the metatarsals in the foot and metacarpals in the hand.
3. Flat bones such as the ilium in the pelvis and parietal in the skull.
4. Irregular bones such cervical vertebrae in the neck and lumbar vertebrae in the lower back.
5. Sesamoid bones such as the patella or knee cap.

The bones of the skeleton are divided into two groups:

1. The axial skeleton (eighty bones).
2. The appendicular skeleton (126 bones).

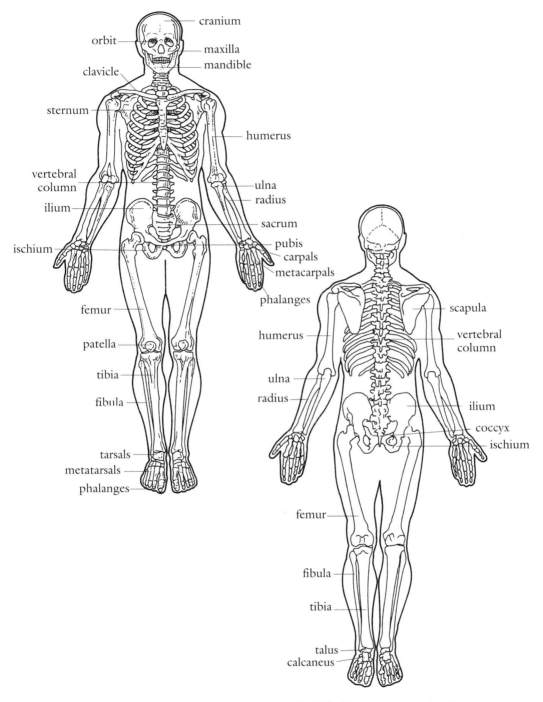

Fig 152. Skeleton – anterior view.

Fig 153. Skeleton – posterior view.

The Axial Skeleton

The axial skeleton consists of the bones of the skull, vertebral column, ribs and sternum.

The skull: These bones are divided into two parts – cranium and face. The bones of the cranium are (Fig 154):

- one frontal bone
- two parietal bones
- two temporal bones
- one occipital bone
- one sphenoid bone
- one ethmoid bone.

The bones of the face are (Fig 155):

- two zygomatic bones
- one maxilla
- two nasal bones
- two lacrimal bones

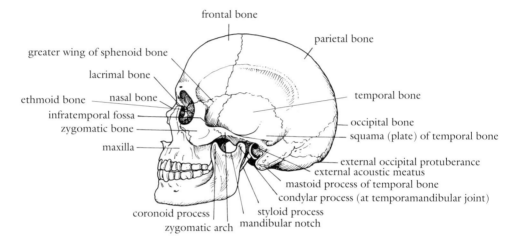

Fig 154. Bones of the cranium.

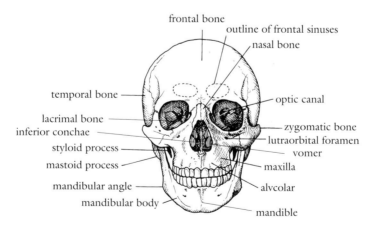

Fig 155. Bones of the face.

- one vomer
- two palatine bones
- two inferior conchae or turbinated bones
- one mandible.

The hyoid bone is an isolated bone lying in the soft tissues of the neck. It does not articulate with any other bone, attaches to the temporal bone by ligaments and gives attachment to the base of the tongue.

The vertebral column: These bones (Fig 156) are divided into twenty-four separate bones in three groups, and the sacrum and coccyx.

The bones of the vertebral column are:

- seven cervical vertebrae
- twelve thoracic vertebrae
- five lumbar vertebrae
- the sacrum – five fused bones
- the coccyx – four fused bones.

The ribs and sternum: These bones (Fig 157) consist of:

- one sternum
- twelve pairs of ribs.

With the twelve thoracic vertebrae, the sternum and ribs form the thorax or thoracic cage.

From the masseur's point of view the most important points to remember are that the first ten pairs of ribs attach at the front (anteriorly) to the sternum by costal cartilages and

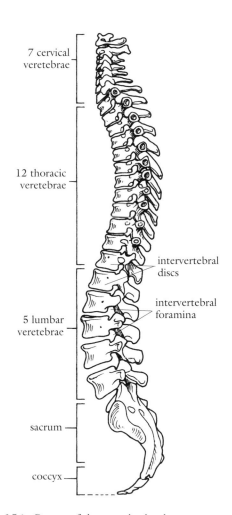

Fig 156. Bones of the vertebral column.

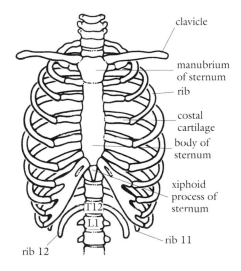

Fig 157. Bones of the ribs and sternum.

the last two pairs of ribs have no anterior attachment. These are often referred to as 'floating ribs'.

The Appendicular Skeleton

The appendicular skeleton (Fig 158) consists of the shoulder girdle and the upper limbs and the pelvic girdle and the lower limbs.

The shoulder girdle: These bones consist of:

- one clavicle (collar bone) each side
- one scapula (shoulder blade) each side.

The upper limb: The bones of the upper limb on each side are:

- one humerus
- one ulna
- one radius
- eight carpal bones
- five metacarpal bones
- fourteen phalanges.

It is important that the sports masseur is aware of the positions of the carpal bones (Fig 159). To be able to name them without reference is a bonus.

The bones of the carpus are divided into two rows:

- proximal row – scaphoid, lunate, triquetral, pisiform
- distal row – trapezium, trapezoid, capitate, hamate.

The pelvic girdle: These bones are:

- two innominate bones, consisting of three fused bones – the ilium, ischium and pubis
- one sacrum.

The landmarks of the innominate bones are

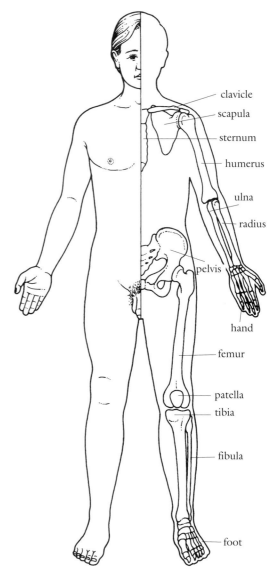

Fig 158. Appendicular skeleton.

extremely useful points for the sports masseur to identify and relate to (Fig 160).

The lower limb: These bones on each side are:

- one femur
- one tibia
- one fibula
- one patella
- seven tarsal bones
- five metatarsal bones
- fourteen phalanges.

The seven tarsal bones (Fig 161) are one talus, one calcaneus, one navicular, three cuneiform and one cuboid.

FUNCTIONS OF THE BONY SKELETON

The skeleton has five principal functions:

1. Support.
2. Movement.
3. Protection.
4. Blood cell production.
5. Calcium storage.

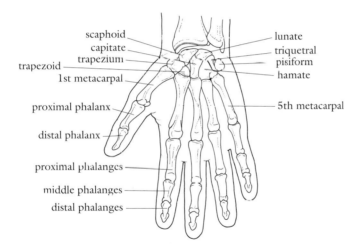

Fig 159. Carpal bones.

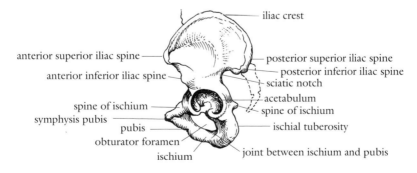

Fig 160. Innominate bone landmarks.

127

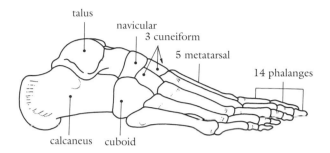

Fig 161. Tarsal bones.

The first three are of major interest to sports masseurs.

Support

The bony skeleton provides the support necessary to maintain upright posture with safety.

Movement

The bones of the skeleton serve as points of attachment for the muscles. The muscles contract and shorten, thus applying force to the bones. The joints between the bones then serve as pivot points that permit movements to take place.

Protection

The bony skeleton forms the outer casing affording protection to the vital, delicate internal organs, such as the brain encased within the skull and the heart and lungs protected by the thorax.

Blood Cell Production

The process of blood cell formation occurs in red bone marrow. Red bone marrow is found in the sternum, ribs and centre of the vertebrae and in the proximal ends of the humerus and femur.

Calcium Storage

The skeleton serves as a massive store, especially of the salts of calcium and phosphorus.

BONE

Bone is the hardest tissue in the body. Bone is composed of one-third organic matrix and two-thirds mineral. The outer, dense layer is called the cortex, and the inner, less dense area is called cancellous bone.

Periosteum

Periosteum almost completely covers bones. It is a vascular fibrous membrane which gives attachment to muscles and tendons and protects the bone from injury. Hyaline cartilage replaces the periosteum on the articular surfaces of synovial joints. Dura mater replaces periosteum on the inner surface of the cranial bones.

Development of Bone

Bone starts to develop before birth and is not complete until about twenty-five years of age. Cartilage models are the forerunners of long, short and irregular bone. Flat bone develops from membrane and sesamoid bones from tendon.

Epiphyses are the extremities of long bone; Diaphysis is the shaft of long bone. Epiphyseal cartilages or growth plates separate the diaphysis from each epiphysis in growing bone. Growth takes place at the diaphyseal surface of these cartilages (Fig 162).

Bony Problems of Import to the Sports Masseur

Fractures: in particular be aware of stress fractures.

Osteoporosis: not just a condition of old age; can be found in sport.

Tumours of the bone: develop for unknown reasons and may be benign or malignant.

Osgood–Schlatter Syndrome: affects the growing tibial tuberosity of adolescents.

Osteochondritis dessicans: most common in the lateral surface of the medial femoral condyle.

JOINTS

Joints are situated where bones meet. There are three classifications of joint:

1. Fibrous – no movement occurs, for example the suture of the skull.
2. Cartilaginous – very slight movement, for example pubic symphysis.
3. Synovial – freely moveable, for example the shoulder joints.

Synovial joints are further classified depending on the ranges of movement possible or the shape of the articular surfaces involved.

Movement at Synovial Joints

Flexion: bending.

Extension: straightening.

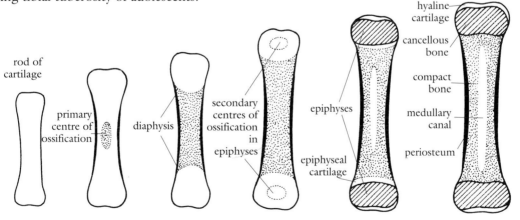

rod of cartilage

primary centre of ossification

diaphysis

secondary centres of ossification in epiphyses

epiphyses

epiphyseal cartilage

hyaline cartilage

cancellous bone

compact bone

medullary canal

periosteum

Fig 162. Development stages of long bones.

Adduction: movement towards the midline or centre of the body.

Abduction: movement away from the midline or centre of the body.

Circumduction: is a circular movement involving flexion, extension, adduction and abduction.

Rotation: turning round on the long axis of a bone: external rotation to the outside, internal rotation to the inside.

Pronation: turning the palm of the hand down.

Supination: turning the palm of the hand up.

Inversion: turning the sole of the foot inward towards the body.

Eversion: turning the sole of the foot outward.

Synovial joints: Ball and socket joint – multi-axial, movement in three planes. These are joints such as the hip and shoulder. The shape of the bones forming the joint allow a wide range of movement. The movements at the ball and socket joint are – flexion, extension, abduction, adduction, rotation and circumduction.

Hinge joint: uniaxial, movement in one plane. These are joints such as the elbow and interphalangeal joints of the fingers and toes. The shape of the bones allow only flexion and extension to take place.

Pivot joint: uniaxial, movement in one plane, rotation. These are joints such as the radioulnar and the joint between the atlas and odontoid process of the axis.

Condyloid joint: biaxial, movement in two planes. Movements are flexion, extension, abduction, adduction and circumduction. These are joints such as the wrist, and metatarsophalangeal.

Gliding joint: the articulating surfaces glide over each other, such as the joints of the tarsus and carpus.

Saddle joint: only found in the thumb; movement as condyloid.

Structure of Synovial Joint (Fig 163)

Articular cartilage: (or hyaline cartilage) covers the parts of the bone ends which form the joint surface.

Joint capsule: (or capsular ligament) a fibrous tissue which surrounds and encloses the joint.

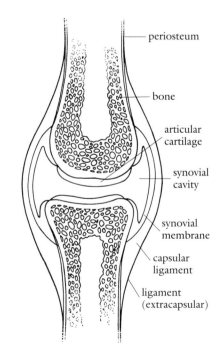

Fig 163. Structure of synovial joint.

Synovial membrane and synovial fluid: lines the capsule, covers those parts of bone within the joint not covered by articular cartilage. The synovial fluid secreted acts as a lubricant.

Joints of the Upper Limb

Joint	Type	Bones	Ligaments	Movements	Muscles
Shoulder	Ball and socket	Humerus	Coracohumeral	Flexion	Coracobrachialis, ant. fibres deltoid, pectoralis major
		Scapula	Glenohumeral		
			Transverse humeral	Extension	Teres major, latissimus dorsi, post. fibres deltoid
				Abduction	Deltoid
				Adduction	Combined action flexors and extensors
				Circumduction	Flexors, extensors abd. and adductors acting in series
				Medial rotation	Pectoralis major, latissimus dorsi, teres major, ant. fibres deltoid
				Lateral rotation	Post. fibres deltoid
Elbow	Hinge	Humerus, ulna	Anterior, posterior, medial, lateral	Flexion	Biceps brachii, brachialis
				Extension	Triceps
Proximal and distal radio-ulnar	Pivot	Radius, ulna	Annular ligament	Pronation	Pronator teres
				Supination	Supinator, biceps
Wrist	Condyloid	Radius, scaphoid lunate, triquetral	Anterior, posterior radio-carpal, medial, lateral	Flexion	Flexor carpi ulnaris, flexor carpi radialis
				Extension	Extensor carpi radialis, longus and brevis, extensor carpi ulnaris
				Abduction	Flexor, extensor carpi radialis
				Adduction	Flexor, extensor carpi ulnaris

131

Bursae: small sacs of synovial fluid found in some joints. These act as a cushion to prevent friction between bone and ligament or tendon or skin.

Menisci or cartilages: found in some joints such as the knee joint. They are made of fibrocartilage and help to stabilize the joint and provide additional cushioning.

Fatty pads: small pads of fat again found in the knee joint. They serve the same purpose as bursae.

Ligaments: attach bone to bone and sometimes blend with the capsule. The ligaments provide stability to the joint.

Muscles or their tendons pass across the joints they move. Nerve and blood supply to the joint capsule and muscles that act upon it, is from the vessels that cross that joint. Muscles contract to move the bone and increase or decrease the joint angle.

Factors Influencing Joint Mobility

- Shape of joint structure.
- Bony structures.
- Effect of muscle groups.
- Periarticular soft structures.
- Temperature.
- Age.
- Sex.

Joints of the Lower Limb

Joint	Type	Bone	Ligaments	Movements	Muscles
Hip	Ball and socket	Innominate, femur	Iliofemoral, ischiofemoral, pubofemoral	Flexion	Iliopsoas, rectus femoris sartorius
				Extension	Gluteus maximus, hamstrings
				Abduction	Gluteus medius, minimus, sartorius, tensor fascia lata
				Adduction	Adductors, gracilis
				External rotation	Gluteals, sartorius, piriformis
				Internal rotation	Gluteus medius, minimus
Knee	Hinge	Femur, tibia	Anterior, posterior cruciates, medial, lateral collateral	Flexion	Hamstrings, gastrocnemius
				Extension	Quadriceps femoris
Ankle	Hinge	Tibia, fibula, talus	Anterior or deltoid, posterior, medial, lateral	Dorsiflexion	Anterior tibials, toe extensors
				Plantarflexion	Gastrocnemius, soleus, toe flexors

Joint Problems of Import to the Sports Masseur

Trauma to the joint: This is usually as result of injury, such as dislocation, sublaxation, soft tissue injury to muscle, ligament, capsule, meniscus, bursa or fatty pad.

Inflammatory disease: These consist of rheumatoid arthritis, polyarthritis or acute infective arthritis.

Osteoarthritis: This is found among many sports people at an earlier age than is usual in the general population.

Connective tissue disease: This tends to occur in early adult life and consists of scleroderma, systemic lupus erythematosus.

MAJOR SYSTEMS – MUSCULAR SYSTEM

There are three types of muscle tissue:

1. Cardiac muscle tissue – found only in the heart.
2. Smooth or involuntary muscle – found in the walls of hollow organs such as the blood and lymph vessels.
3. Skeletal or voluntary muscle – found in the muscles used to move the joints.

The Skeletal Muscle

For our purpose we shall address the skeletal muscle only (Figs 164, 165 & 166).

- Each muscle fibre has several nuclei just under the sarcolemma or cell membrane.
- Muscle fibres lie parallel to one another.
- Sarcomere is the individual contractile unit and consists of thin filaments of actin and thick filaments of myosin.
- Endomysium is a fine meshwork of loose connective tissue surrounding each muscle fibre.
- Fasciculi are groups of fifteen to forty fibres bound into bundles.
- Perimyseum is a coarse fibrous connective tissue sheath covering each fasicle.

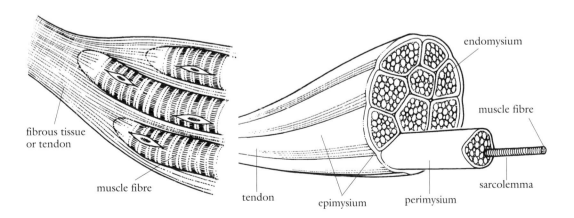

Fig 164. Skeletal muscle fibre and connective tissue.

Fig 165. Cross-section skeletal muscle fibre.

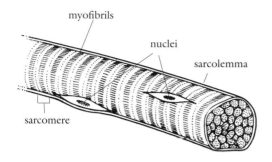

Fig 166. Single muscle fibre.

- Epimysium is the thicker outer connective tissue sheath.
- Tendon attaches muscle to bone or skin. This is made up of the epimysium, perimysium and endomysium becoming continuous with fibrous tissue that extends from the muscle.

Blood brings oxygen and food to muscles and carries away the waste products produced by muscular contraction. Muscles cannot function without a continuous supply of food and removal of waste. The energy source required for muscle contraction is ATP – adenosine triphosphate. This chemical energy is produced from glucose and oxygen by cellular oxidation. Glycogen is a carbohydrate store which is broken down into glucose when required. Myoglobin is a unique oxygen binding protein molecule which stores oxygen inside the muscle cells. Phosphocreatine (PC) is stored in the muscle and is broken down into phosphorus and creatine.

Muscle Fibre Types

The two major fibre types are type 1 – fast twitch fibres and type 2 – slow twitch fibres. The fast twitch, type 1 fibres are adapted to function for power/strength activities. The slow twitch, type 2 fibres are adapted for endurance activities.

Muscle Action

Four headings are used to identify each muscle's function:

Agonist or prime mover: The muscle or muscles whose contraction actually produces movement, such as elbow flexion, biceps.

Antagonist: The muscle or muscles which oppose the action of another muscle, for example elbow flexion, is opposed by triceps.

Fixator: Stabilizes bones from which the prime movers originate, for example abducting the arm, the muscles of the shoulder girdle.

Synergist: Muscle which contracts at the same time as the prime mover, assisting or supplementing the movement produced, for example internal, external abdominal obliques.

There are five types of muscle action:

Concentric contraction: The muscle shortens, bringing origin and insertion closer together. The joint angle decreases.

Eccentric contraction: The muscle lengthens. Origin and insertion move further apart and there is an increase in the joint angle.

Isotonic contraction: The muscle is tensioned to overcome a resistance and there is joint movement.

Isometric contraction: Often called static contraction The muscle is tensioned but there is no movement of the joint.

Isokinetic contraction: The muscle contracts at a constant speed over the full range of the movement.

Muscles are attached to bones by tendons. The origin is the muscle attachment which remains stationary when the muscle contracts, for example biceps to scapula. The insertion is the muscle attachment which moves when the muscle contracts, for example biceps to radius.

Muscles Acting on the Neck

Muscle	Origin	Insertion	Function	Nerve Supply
Sternocleido-mastoid	Sternum, clavicle	Temporal bone	Flexion/rotation	Accessory nerve
Semispinalis capitis	Lower four cervical, Upper six thoracic vertebrae	Occipital bone	Extension/lateral	First five cervical nerves

Muscles Acting on the Chest Wall

Muscle	Origin	Insertion	Function	Nerve Supply
External intercostals	Rib lower border	Rib upper border (rib below origin)	Elevate ribs	Intercostal nerves
Internal intercostals	Rib, inner surface lower border	Rib upper border (rib below origin)	Depress ribs	Intercostal nerves
Diaphragm	Lower circumference of thorax	Central tendon of diaphragm	Enlarges thorax causing inspiration	Phrenic nerves

Muscles Acting on the Abdominal Wall

Muscle	Origin	Insertion	Function	Nerve Supply
External oblique	Lower eight ribs	Ossa coxae Linea alba	Compresses abdomen Important postural muscle pulling front of pelvis up	Lower seven intercostal nerves
Internal oblique	Ossa coxae	Ribs, public bone, linea alba	As above	Last three intercostal nerves
Transversalis	Ribs, Ossa coxae	Pubic bone, Linea alba	As external oblique	Last five intercostal nerves
Rectus abdominus	Pubic bone, pubic symphysis	Costal cartilage five, six, seven ribs Sternum	As above Flexes trunk	Last six intercostal nerves

Muscles Acting on the Trunk

Muscle	Origin	Insertion	Action	Nerve Supply
Sacrospinalis	Iliac crest, ribs Vertebrae	Ribs, vertebrae Temporal bone	Extends spine Abducts and rotates trunk	First cervical to fifth lumbar spinal nerve
Quadratus lumborum	Ilium – posterior crest Lumbar vertebrae three to five	Twelfth ribs Lumbar vertebrae one to four	Extends and abducts spine	First three lumbar nerves
Iliopsoas	Ilium – iliac fossa	Femur – lesser trochanter	Flexes trunk	Femoral, second to fourth lumbar

Muscles Acting on the Shoulder

Muscle	Origin	Insertion	Action	Nerve Supply
Trapezius	Occipital bone Cervical, thoracic vertebrae	Clavicle	Depresses, elevates shoulders, extends head	Cervical nerves two to four
Serratus Anterior	Ribs – upper nine	Scapula – anterior vertebral border	Abduction, external, Anterior depression of shoulder	Long thoracic nerve
Pectoralis minor	Ribs two to five	Coracoid	Anterior depression of shoulder	Med., lat., ant. thoracic nerve

Muscles Acting on the Upper Arm

Muscle	Origin	Insertion	Action	Nerve Supply
Pectoralis major	Clavicle, sternum	Humerus – greater tubercle	Flexion, adduction	Med., lat., ant. thoracic nerve
Latissimus dorsi	Spines of lower thoracic and lumbar vertebrae and posterior iliac crest	Bicipital groove of humerus	Adduction, med. rotation and extension	Thoracodorsal nerve
Deltoid	Clavicle and scapula	Deltoid tuberosity of humerus	Anterior fibres flexion, middle fibres abduction, posterior fibres extension	Axillary nerve
Coracobrachialis	Coracoid process of scapula	Middle third of humerus	Adduction, internal rotation	Musculocutaneous nerve
Supraspinatus	Scapula supraspinous fossa	Greater tubercle of humerus	Abduction	Suprascapular nerve

Muscles Acting on the Upper Arm *continued*

Muscle	Origin	Insertion	Action	Nerve Supply
Infraspinatus	Scapula infraspinous border	Greater tubercle of humerus	External rotation	Suprascapular nerve
Teres major	Axillary border of scapula	Upper anterior of humerus	Extension adduction internal rotation	Lower subscapular nerve
Teres minor	Axillary border of scapula	Greater tubercle of humerus	External rotation	Axillary nerve

Muscles Acting on the Lower Arm

Muscle	Origin	Insertion	Action	Nerve Supply
Biceps brachii	Scapula supraglenoid tuberosity and coracoid	Tubercle of radius proximal end	Flexes supinated forearm supinates forearm	Musculocutaneous nerve
Brachialis	Ant. surface distal half humerus	Coronocoid process of ulna	Flexes pronated forearm	Musculocutaneous nerve
Brachioradialis	Lateral epicondyle of humerus	Styloid process of radius	Flexes semi-pronated or semisupinated forearm supinates forearm	Radial nerve
Triceps brachii	Scapula, medial and lateral heads from humerus	Olecranon process of ulna	Extends lower arm	Radial nerve
Pronator teres	Med. condyle humerus coronoid process ulna	Middle third radius	Pronates and flexes forearm	Median nerve
Pronator quadratus	Distal part of ulna	Distal part radius	Pronates forearm	Median nerve
Supinator	Lateral epicondyle humerus Proximal part of ulna	Radius proximal part	Supinates forearm	Radial nerve

Muscles Acting on the Hand

Muscle	Origin	Insertion	Action	Nerve Supply
Extensor carpi ulnaris	Lateral epicondyle humerus Proximal part of ulna	Fifth metacarpal	Extends, adducts hand	Radial nerve
Extensor carpi radialis brevis	Lateral epicondyle humerus	Second, third metacarpals	Extends hand	Radial nerve

Muscles Acting on the Hand *continued*

Muscle	Origin	Insertion	Action	Nerve Supply
Extensor carpi radialis longus	Above lateral epicondyle humerus	Second metacarpal	Extends, abducts hand	Radial nerve
Palmaris longus	Medial epicondyle humerus	Fascia of palm	Flexes hand	Median nerve
Flexor carpi ulnaris	Medial epicondyle humerus proximal part ulna	Pisiform, third, fourth fifth metacarpals	Flexes, adducts hand	Ulnar nerve
Flexor carpi radialis	Medial epicondyle humerus	Second metacarpal	Flexes forearm, hand	Median nerve

Muscles Acting on the Thigh

Muscle	Origin	Insertion	Action	Nerve Supply
Iliopsoas	Iliac fossa, twelfth thoracic to fifth lumbar vertebrae	Lesser trochanter femur	Flexes thigh and trunk	Femoral, two to four lumbar nerves
Rectus femoris	Anterior inferior iliac spine	Tibial tuberosity	Flexes thigh, extends lower leg	Femoral nerve
Gluteus maximus	Iliac crest, sacrum, coccyx	Greater trochanter femur iliotibial tract	Extends and external rotation	Inferior gluteal nerve
Gluteus medius	Lateral surface ilium	Greater trochanter femur	Abducts and internal rotation	Superior gluteal nerve
Gluteus minimus	Lateral surface ilium	Greater trochanter femur	As medius	As medius
Tensor fascia lata	Anterior iliac crest	Tibia by iliotibial tract	Abducts, tightens iliotibial tract	As medius
Piriformis	Anterior sacrum	Medial part greater trochanter femur	Abducts, extends, external rotation	First or second sacral nerve
Adductor brevis	Pubic bone	Linea aspera femur	Adducts	Obturator nerve
Adductor longus	As brevis	As brevis	As brevis	As brevis
Adductor magnus	As brevis	As brevis	As brevis	As brevis
Gracilis	Below symphysis pubic bone	Medial surface tibia	Adducts, flexes	Obturator nerve

Muscles Acting on the Lower Leg

Muscle	Origin	Insertion	Action	Nerve Supply
Rectus femoris	Anterior inferior iliac spine	Tibial tuberosity	Flexes thigh, extends knee	Femoral nerve

Muscles Acting on the Lower Leg *continued*

Muscle	Origin	Insertion	Action	Nerve Supply
Vastus lateralis	Linea aspera of femur	As rectus	Extends knee	As rectus
Vastus medialis	Femur	As rectus	As lateralis	As rectus
Vastus intermedius	Anterior aspect femur	As rectus	As lateralis	As rectus
Sartorius	Anterior superior iliac spine	Medial surface upper end tibia	Adducts, flexes leg	Femoral nerve
Biceps femoris	Ischial tuberosity Linea aspera femur	Head of fibula lateral condyle tibia	Flexes knee Extends thigh	Branch of sciatic nerve
Semitendinosus	As biceps femoris	Tibia proximal end medial surface	As biceps femoris	As biceps femoris
Semimembranosus	Ischial tuberosity	Medial condyle tibia	As biceps femoris	As biceps femoris

Muscles Acting on Foot and Ankle

Muscle	Origin	Insertion	Action	Nerve Supply
Tibialis anterior	Lateral condyle tibia	Cunieform, base first metatarsal	Dorsiflexion inversion	Common and deep
Gastrocnemius	Medial and lateral femoral condyles	Calcaneus – forms tendo achilles	Plantar flexion flexes lower leg	Tibial nerve
Soleus	Tibia, fibula (deep to gastrocnemius)	Calcaneus via tendo achilles	Plantar flexion	As gastrocnemius
Peroneus longus	Lateral condyle tibia, head of fibula	Cunieform, base of first metatarsal	Plantar flexion eversion	Common peroneal nerve
Peroneus brevis	Lower lateral shaft fibula	Fifth metatarsal	Eversion, dorsiflexion	Superficial peroneal nerve
Peroneus tertius	Distal third fibula	Fourth, fifth metatarsals	Eversion, dorsiflexion	Deep peroneal nerve
Tibialis posterior	Posterior tibial, posterior fibula	Cuboid, navicular, cunieforms, second and fourth metatarsals	Plantar flexion inversion	Tibial nerve
Popliteus	Lateral femoral condyle	Soleal line of tibia	Flexes, medially rotates	Medial popliteal nerve

Muscles Acting on the Fingers

Muscle	Origin	Insertion	Action	Nerve Supply
Extensor digitorum	Lateral epicondyle humerus	Bases middle, distal phalanges	Extends phalanges and hand	Posterior interosseous

Muscles Acting on the Fingers *continued*

Muscle	Origin	Insertion	Action	Nerve Supply
Extensor minimi digiti	As digitorum	Second and third phalanges	As digitorum	As digitorum
Abductor pollicis longus	Ulna, radius, interosseus membrane	Base of first metacarpal	Abducts thumb, extends hand	As digitorum
Extensor pollicis brevis	Radius, interosseous membrane	Base proximal phalanx of thumb	Extends proximal phalanx, extends, abducts hand	Posterior interosseous
Extensor pollicis longus	Ulna, interosseous membrane	Base of distal phalanx of thumb	Extends phalanges and metacarpal of thumb, extends, abducts hand	As brevis
Extensor indicis	As pollicis longus	Tendon of digitorum	Extends index finger, hand	As brevis
Flexor digitorum sublimus	Medial epicondyle, radial head	Margins of middle phalanx	Flexes middle and proximal phalanges and wrist	Median nerve
Flexor digitorum profundus	Ulna, interosseous membrane	Palmar surface base of distal phalanx	Flexes all three phalanges and wrist	Anterior interosseous
Lumbricales (four muscles)	Tendons of flexor profundus	Extensor tendons of fingers base proximal phalanx and joint capsule	Flexes proximal phalanx, extends other two phalanges	Median – first/ second Ulnar – third/fourth
Flexor pollicis longus	Radius, interosseous membrane	Base distal phalanx thumb	Flexes thumb	Median nerve
Flexor pollicis brevis	Flexor retinaculum	Proximal phalanx of thumb	Flexes thumb	Median nerve
Abductor pollicis brevis	Flexor retinaculum scaphoid, trapezium	As above	Abducts carpo-metacarpal joint	As above
Adductor pollicis	Carpus, metacarpals	As above	Adducts thumb	As above
Opponens pollicis	Flexor retinaculum, trapezium	Metacarpal of thumb	Flexes meta-carpal, rotates it medially	As above

Muscles Acting on the Toes

Muscle	Origin	Insertion	Action	Nerve Supply
Extensor digitorum longus	Upper fibula	Middle and distal phalanges of lateral four toes	Extends toes, dorsiflexes foot	Anterior tibial nerve
Extensor digitorum brevis	Inferior extensor retinaculum, calcaneum	Proximal phalanx big toe, tendons extensor expansions	Extends meta-tarso phalangial joint	As above
Extensor hallucis longus	Fibula	Distal phalanx big toe	Extends big toe, dorsiflexes foot	As above
Abductor hallucis	Flexor retinaculum, calcaneum	Proximal phalanx big toe	Abducts, flexes big toe	Medial plantar nerve
Abductor digiti minimi	Calcaneum	Proximal phalanx little toe	Abducts, flexes little toe	Lateral plantar nerve
Flexor digitorum brevis	Calcaneum	Middle phalanges	Flexes middle, proximal phalanges	Medial plantar nerve
Flexor digitorum longus	Tibia	Base of distal phalanges	Flexes toes, plantar flex foot	Posterior tibial
Flexor hallucis longus	Fibula	Distal phalanx big toe	Flexes big toe plantar flexes foot	As above
Lumbricals (four muscles)	First – tendon long flexor Second to fourth – tendons flexor longus	Extensor tendons proximal phalanges, joint capsule nerve	Flexes proximal phalanges Extends middle and distal	First medial plantar nerve Two to four lateral plantar nerve
Flexor hallucis brevis	Cuboid, cunieform	Proximal phalanx	Flexes big toe	Medial plantar nerve
Adductor hallucis	Peroneus longus sheath, two to four metatarsals, lateral four plantar ligaments	As above	Adducts and flexes toes	Lateral plantar nerve
Flexor digiti minimi	Peroneus longus, fifth metatarsal	Proximal phalanx little toe	Flexes little toe	As above
Plantar interossei (three muscles)	Three to five metatarsals	Three to five toes	Flex proximal, extend middle distal phalanges, adduct toes	Lateral plantar nerve
Dorsal interossei (four muscles)	Metatarsals	Toes	Flex, extend as above, abduct toes	As above

MAJOR SYSTEMS – VASCULAR SYSTEM

The vascular system consists of:

1. The heart
2. Blood vessels
3. Blood

The Heart

The heart is a muscular organ divided into four chambers (Fig 167): the right atrium, left atrium, right ventricle, and left ventricle.

- Venous blood is in the right side of the heart, arterial blood is in the left side. The right side is separated from the left side by a septum to prevent venous blood contacting arterial blood.

- The right atrium receives blood from the body via the superior and inferior vena cavae and the coronary sinus.
- The left atrium receives blood from the lungs via the pulmonary veins.
- The right ventricle sends blood to the lungs via the pulmonary artery.
- The left ventricle sends blood to the body via the aorta.
- The mitral valve prevents backflow from the left ventricle.
- The tricuspid valve prevents backflow from the right ventricle.
- The semilunar valves prevent backflow from the pulmonary artery and the aorta.
- The pulmonary circulation takes blood from the right ventricle to the lungs, and returns blood to the left atrium.
- The systemic circulation takes blood around the body from the left ventricle,

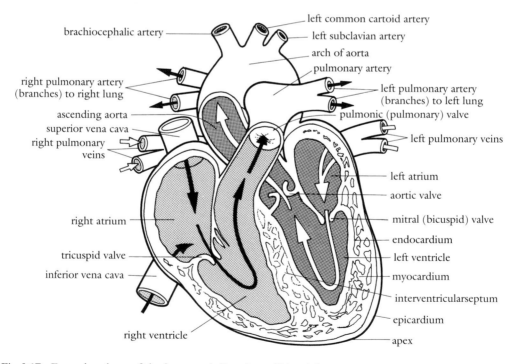

Fig 167. Four chambers of the heart and direction of blood flow.

and returns blood to the right atrium.

- Contraction of the heart muscle is called systole.
- Relaxation of the heart muscle is called diastole.

Blood Vessels

- Blood is taken from the heart by arteries and arterioles.
- Blood is returned to the heart by veins and venules.
- Arterial blood is oxygenated, venous blood is deoxygenated.
- Capillaries carry a mixture of oxygenated and deoxygenated blood.
- The aorta is the largest artery in the body.
- The walls of veins are thinner than the walls of arteries.

Blood

- There are five to six litres of blood circulating in the average adult.
- Blood consists of: plasma; erythrocytes or red corpuscles; leucocytes or white corpuscles; thrombocytes or platelets.
- Plasma is the liquid basis of the blood and is a clear yellowish fluid.
- Erythrocytes contain haemoglobin which gives them their colour. Haemoglobin has the ability to absorb oxygen. Erythrocytes are produced in red bone marrow.
- Leukocytes are larger than erythrocytes. Their main role is to protect the body from infection and their numbers increase when infections occur. They are produced in bone marrow.
- Thrombocytes are essential to the clotting or coagulation of blood. They are produced in bone marrow.
- Normal pulse rate of 60–100 beats per minute is often lower in sports participants.

MAJOR SYSTEMS – LYMPHATIC SYSTEM

The lymphatic system returns plasma proteins and tissue fluid to the blood. This system is involved in the specific and non-specific defence mechanisms of the body. The constituents of the lymphatic system are: lymph vessels; lymph nodes; spleen; thymus gland.

Lymph Vessels

- Lymph capillaries originate as blind-end tubes in the interstitial tissue. Their walls are more permeable to all interstitial fluid particles including proteins and cell debris than are the walls of blood capillaries. The tiny lymph capillaries join up to form the larger lymph vessels. Lymph vessels have numerous semilunar valves to ensure that lymph will only flow towards the thorax.
- The muscle tissue within the walls of these vessels contracts to move the lymph on.
- Contraction of surrounding muscle, tissue fluid pressure, pulsation of adjacent arteries causing pressure and the negative pressure in the thorax during inspiration, all have effects on lymph flow.
- Lymph vessels join up to form two large ducts – the thoracic duct and the right lymphatic duct. Both empty lymph into the subclavian veins.
- The thoracic duct drains lymph from both legs, pelvic and abdominal cavities, left half of the thorax, left arm, left side of the head and neck.
- The right lymphatic duct drains the lymph from the right arm, right half of the thorax, and right side of the head and neck.

Functions of Lymph Vessels

- Return plasma proteins to the blood.
- Return excess tissue fluid to the blood.

- Transport cell debris and micro-organisms from the tissues to the lymph nodes for breakdown.
- Fat absorbed in the small intestine is carried via the lymph system to the thoracic duct.

Lymph Nodes

Lymph drains through the lymph nodes before returning to the blood. These nodes vary in size from tiny – pinhead size to about 3cm (1¼in) in length. They are strategically situated:

- Lymph from the head and neck passes through deep and superficial cervical nodes, situated in the neck (Fig 168).
- Lymph from the arms passes through the nodes in the elbow area and then the superficial and deep axillary nodes (Fig 169).
- Lymph from the legs passes through the deep and superficial nodes situated behind the knee (popliteal nodes) and groin (inguinal nodes) (Fig 170).
- Lymph from the internal organs, pelvis and abdomen drains into nodes closely related to their blood vessels and eventually drains into the cisterna chyli.

Spleen

The spleen is situated in the upper left abdominal cavity (Fig 171). The function of the spleen is to destroy old and abnormal erythrocytes. The spleen supplies many of the erythtocytes in the blood.

Thymus Gland

This gland is situated in the upper part of the chest behind the sternum and extends into the neck. Lymphocytes which originate in

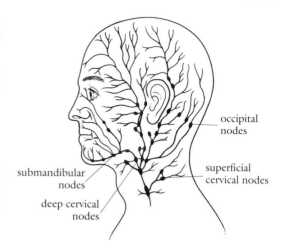

Fig 168. Lymph nodes of the neck.

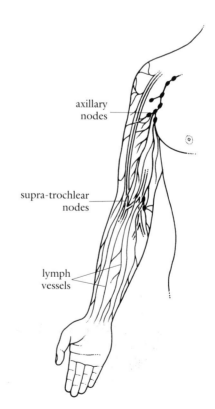

Fig 169. Axillary lymph nodes.

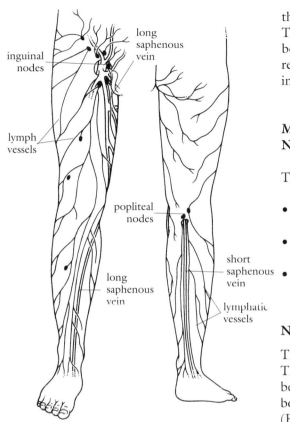

Fig 170. Leg lymph nodes.

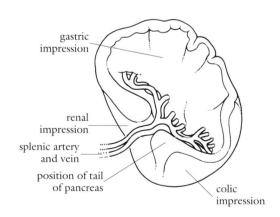

Fig 171. Spleen.

the red bone marrow may enter the thymus. Those lymphocytes which do mature become activated T-lymphocytes, which respond to antigens encountered elsewhere in the body.

MAJOR SYSTEMS – NEUROLOGICAL SYSTEM

This system is best revised as:

- The central nervous system, which consists of the brain and spinal cord.
- The peripheral nervous system, which consists of thirty-one pairs of spinal nerves.
- The autonomic nervous system, which consists of twelve pairs of cranial nerves.

Neurones

These are commonly referred to as nerves. The nervous system consists of a large number of these neurones. Each neurone has a cell body and its processes – axons and dendrites (Fig 172). Neurones have the ability to display conductivity or irritability. Neurones synthesise A.T.P. from glucose.

Conductivity

Conductivity is the ability to transmit an impulse. This impulse may be from one part of the brain to another. An impulse from the brain to a muscle results in voluntary muscle contraction. These impulses are also responsible for balance, posture, secretion of glands, and regulation of body function. Sensory nerve endings also use impulses to alert the brain to temperature, touch and pain. Communications from the outside world through the organs of sense, such as ears, nose, eyes and tongue, are delivered by impulse.

145

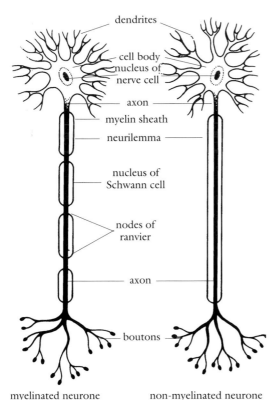

dendrites
cell body
nucleus of nerve cell
axon
myelin sheath
neurilemma
nucleus of Schwann cell
nodes of ranvier
axon
boutons

myelinated neurone   non-myelinated neurone

Fig 172. Neurone.

Irritability

Irritability is the ability to initiate nerve impulses in response to stimuli both from inside and outside the body, for example inside the body a thought can result in a voluntary movement, outside touch results in a reaction.

Ganglion

The ganglion is a group of nerve cell bodies, usually found outside the central nervous system.

The Peripheral Nervous System

This consists of afferent and efferent divisions. Afferent or sensory nerves carry impulses from the sensory nerve endings to the central nervous system. Efferent or motor nerves carry impulses from the central nervous system to the effector organs, that is glands and muscles.

The efferent division is further divided into the autonomic nervous system and the somatic nervous system. The autonomic or involuntary nervous system transmits from the central nervous system to smooth muscle such as cardiac muscle. The somatic nervous system transmits from the central nervous system to the skeletal muscles.

The autonomic nervous system is divided into the sympathetic and the parasympathetic systems. The sympathetic nervous system conveys impulses from the central nervous system to the effector organs and tissues, such as the stomach, intestines and salivary glands. These impulses are associated with preparing the organs for action. The parasympathetic nervous system is involved with similar organs but in the resting state, such as food digestion and absorption.

The Central Nervous System

This consists of the brain and spinal column. This system is responsible for mental activities, sensory perception, initiation and control of voluntary muscle contraction.

MINOR SYSTEMS – DIGESTIVE SYSTEM

Digestive system is the name given to the system which deals with changing the food taken into the body. The food is converted into nutrients, which are absorbed into the blood-

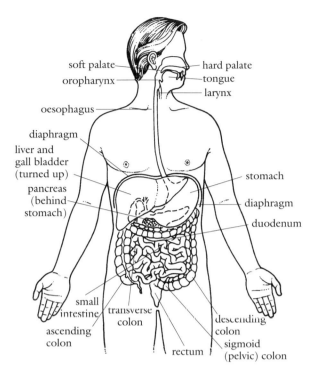

soft palate
oropharynx

hard palate
tongue
larynx

oesophagus

diaphragm
liver and
gall bladder
(turned up)
pancreas
(behind
stomach)

stomach

diaphragm

duodenum

small
intestine
transverse
colon
ascending
colon

descending
colon
sigmoid
(pelvic) colon
rectum

Fig 173. Organs of the digestive system.

stream and the indigestible remnants are then evacuated (Fig 173). The main components of the digestive tract are:

Alimentary canal: mouth, pharynx, oesophagus, stomach, small intestine, large intestine, rectum and anal canal.

Accessory organs: three pairs of salivary glands, pancreas, liver and the biliary tract.

Metabolism

Metabolism is the term used to refer to all the chemical reactions that occur in the body. Absorbed nutrients are used to provide energy and to make new or replacement body substances. Catabolism breaks down large molecules and abolism builds up large molecules.

MINOR SYSTEMS – RESPIRATORY SYSTEM

The respiratory system takes in oxygen and excretes carbon dioxide. The organs of the respiratory system are: nose, pharynx, larynx, trachea, two bronchi, bronchioles, alveoli, two lungs, pleura, and muscles of respiration (intercostal muscles and the diaphragm). (Fig 174).

- Taking air into the body is known as Inspiration, excreting air from the body is known as Expiration.
- Respiration is the name given to the movement of gases from the air to the tissues and their return by the blood.
- Ventilation is part of respiration and deals with the mechanics of moving air into and out of the lungs.

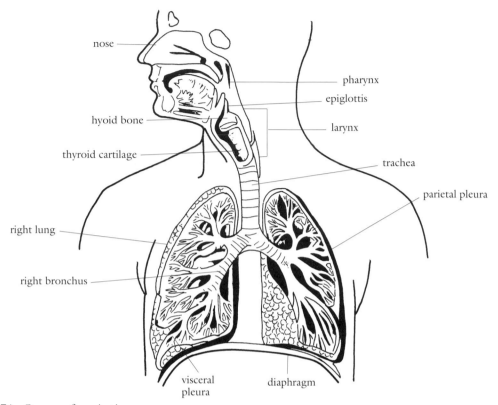

nose

pharynx

epiglottis

hyoid bone

larynx

thyroid cartilage

trachea

parietal pleura

right lung

right bronchus

visceral pleura

diaphragm

Fig 174. Organs of respiration.

- Internal respiration is the exchange of gases between tissue cells and the interstitial fluid.
- External respiration is the exchange of gases between the body and the external environment.
- Exercise induced asthma is fairly common in sport. This condition restricts expiration.

MINOR SYSTEMS – GENITO-URINARY SYSTEM

This system consists of the reproductive system and the excretory system. The reproductive system is dealt with as the female system and the male system.

The Female Reproductive System

This consists of external genitalia and internal organs.

External genitalia or vulva: These consist of the labia majora, labia minora, clitoris, vestibule and greater vestibular glands (Fig 175).

Internal organs: These consist of the vagina, uterus, two uterine tubes and two ovaries (Fig 176).

The functions of the female reproductive system are:

- Formation of ova.
- Reception of spermatozoa.
- Provision of a suitable environment for fertilization.

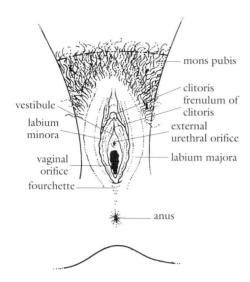

Fig 175. External genitalia of the female.

- Provision of a suitable environment for development of the fetus.
- Childbirth.

The Male Reproductive System

This consists of two testes and two epididymides in the scrotum, two vas deferens, two spermatic cords, two seminal vesicles, two ejaculatory ducts, one prostate gland and one penis (Fig 177).

The functions of the male reproductive system are:

- Production of spermatozoa.
- Transmission of spermatozoa to the female.

The Urinary or Excretory System

This consists of two kidneys, two ureters, one urinary bladder and one urethra (Fig 178).

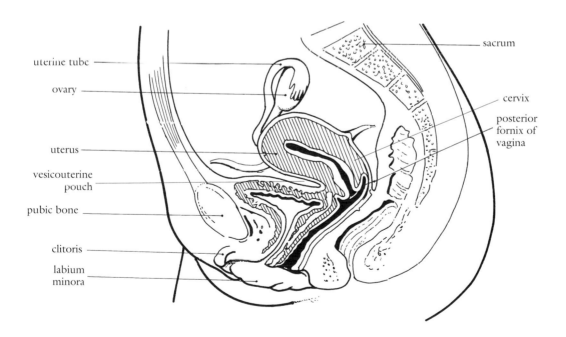

Fig 176. Internal genital organs of the female.

149

Fig 177. Male reproductive organs.

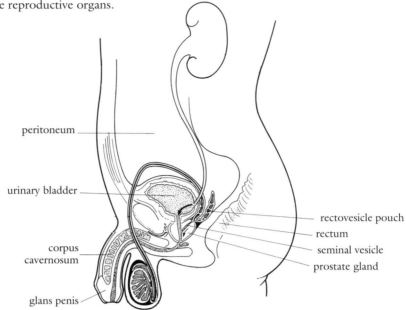

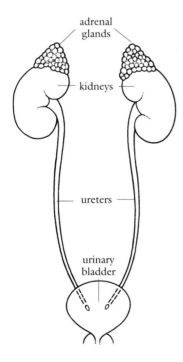

Fig 178. Ureters, kidney and bladder.

The function of the urinary system is:

- The kidneys maintain the purity and constancy of fluids and secrete urine.
- The ureters take the urine from the kidneys to the urinary bladder.
- The urinary bladder is where urine collects and is temporarily stored.
- The urethra excretes urine from the urinary bladder to the exterior. Micturition or urination is the act of emptying the bladder.

MINOR SYSTEMS – ENDOCRINE SYSTEM

The endocrine system consists of a number of glands which secrete hormones (Fig 179). This system consists of one pituitary gland, one thyroid gland, four parathyroid glands, two adrenal or suprarenal glands, the pancreatic islets, one pineal gland, one thymus gland, two ovaries in the female and two

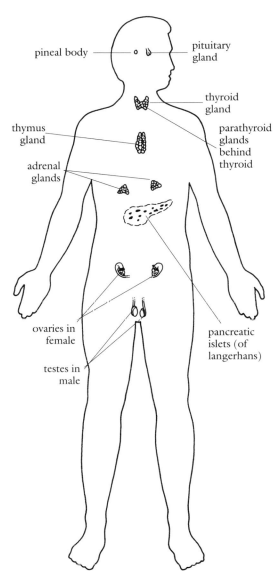

THE SKIN

The other body structure which is of importance to the masseur is the skin. It is not regarded as a major or minor body system but rather as a protective system. The skin consists of two main layers:

- The epidermis or outer skin (Fig 180).
- The dermis or under layer (Fig 181).

The Epidermis

This consists of four strata:

- Germinative layer – the deepest layer.
- Stratum granulosum.
- Stratum lucidum.
- Stratum corneum – surface layer.

Fig 179. Position of endocrine glands.

testes in the male. Hormones are secreted by the glands of the endocrine system. A hormone is a chemical messenger, which is formed in one gland and then travels via the blood to another organ where it influences activity, nutrition and growth.

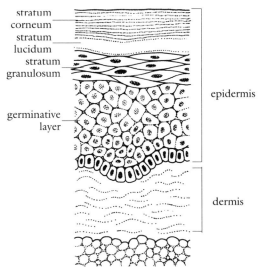

Fig 180. Epidermis.

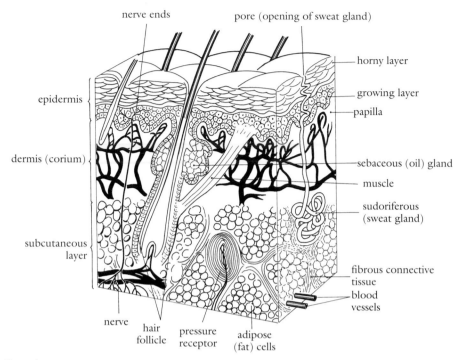

Fig 181. Dermis.

The function of the skin is:

- To protect the underlying structures from injury.
- To protect the underlying structures from entry by germs.
- To protect the body from water loss.
- To be part of temperature regulation.
- To contain nerve endings for sensing pain, temperature and touch.

As previously stated, the condition of skin is very important to the masseur and can often be the reason why massage is not applied. For example, as well as skin infections, allergies, pressure sores, burns and cuts, the masseur should always be aware of any skin tumours. These may well be benign but some can be malignant. It is as usual good practice to alert the participant of any skin condition which is present and refer on to the appropriate professional.

Bibliography

Arnheim, Daniel D. (1986), *Dance Injuries*, Princeton Book Company, Pennington.

Arnould-Taylor, W.E. (1977), *The Principles and Practice of Physical Therapy*, Stanley Thomas, London.

Athletic Training and Sports Medicines (1985), The American Academy of Orthopaedic Surgeons, Illinois.

Australian Family Physician (1982), Biersdorf Australia Ltd.

Beard, G. (1974), *Massage Principles and Techniques*, Saunders, Philidelphia.

Booher, James M. and Thibodeau, Gary A. (1983), *Athletic Injury Assessment*, Times Mirror/Mosby College Publishing, St Louis.

Cash, Mel (1996), *Sports and Remedial Massage Therapy*, Ebury Press, London.

Cyriax, J.U. (1977), *Textbook of Orthopaedic Medicine*, Vol 2, Balliere Tindall, London.

Downer, Jane (1992), *Shiatsu*, Hodder & Stoughton Ltd, Sevenoaks.

Holey, Elizabeth and Cook, Eileen (1977), *Therapeutic Massage*, W.B. Saunders Co. Ltd, London.

Hollis, Margaret (1987), *Massage for Therapists*, Blackwell Science, Oxford.

Hollis, Margaret (1998), *Massage for Therapists*, Second edition, Blackwell Science, Oxford.

Jarmey, Chris and Tindall, John (1991), *Acupressure for Common Ailments*, Gaia Books, London.

Ross and Wilson (1996), *Anatomy and Physiology*, Churchill Livingstone, Edinburgh.

Ryman, Daniele (1984), *The Aromatherapy Handbook*, Century Publishing Co., Great Britain.

Stomer, Chris (1996), *Teach Yourself Reflexology*, Hodder Headline Plc, London.

Wallis, E.L. and Logan G.A. (1964), *Figure Improvement and Body Conditioning Through Exercise*, Prentice Hall, New York.

Williams, J. (1974), *Massage and Sport*, Bayer, Switzerland.

Yalin, J. and Cash, M. (1988) *Sports Massage*, Stanley Paul, London.

Glossary

Abduction – Movement of limb away from the midline.

Adduction – Movement of limb towards the midline.

Agonist – Muscle directly engaged in contraction.

Anatomy – Study of the structure of the body and relationship of the various components to each other.

Angina – Chest pain, caused by lack of oxygen for the heart.

Antagonist – Muscle which counteracts the action of another muscle.

Anterior – Front part of the body.

Arteriosclerosis – A disease characterized by thickening and loss of elasticity of the arterial walls.

Articular – Pertaining to a joint.

Astringent – Lotion that closes skin pores.

A.T.P. – Adenosine Triphosphate.

Atrium – Either of the two upper chambers of the heart.

Bilateral – On both sides.

Blood pressure – Pressure of the blood against the walls of the arteries as it passes through.

Bronchi – Branches of the trachea that lead into the lungs.

Capsule – Fibrous tissues enclosing a joint.

Cardiovascular system – Heart and blood vessels.

Centrifugal – Away from the heart.

Centripetal – Towards the heart.

Cervical spine – Seven bones found in the neck.

Conditioning – Exercising the body for a specific task.

CTM – Connective tissue massage.

Dermis – The inner layer of the skin.

Diabetis mellitus – Disease in which the body is unable to use sugar usually because of insulin deficiency.

Diagnosis – Identification of a disease or injury from its signs and symptoms.

Diaphysis – Shaft of long bone.

Dilate – Swell.

Distal – Furthest from the centre.

Dominant side – Side of preference, for example right-handed.

Dorsal – Behind.

Dorsal spine – Thoracic spine.

Dorsiflexion – Action of a joint towards the posterior surface.

Dysfunction – Abnormal function.

Effusion – Swelling of joint.

Epicondyle – Eminences on side of bone.

Epiphyseal plate – Cartilage plate near the end of a child's bone, where growth takes place.

Epiphysis – End of long bone.

Eversion – Turning out.

Extend – To straighten a joint.

Extremities – Arms and legs.

Flexion – Bending a joint.

Genitalia – Male and female reproductive systems.

Haematoma – Pool of blood collected within damaged tissue.

Haemophilia – Hereditary bleeding disorder.

Haemorrhage – Bleeding.

Hamstring – Muscle group at the back of the

thigh.

Hypertension – Abnormally and persistently high blood pressure.

Innominate bone – Bone forming one half of the pelvic girdle.

Insertion – Site of attachment of muscle.

Lateral – Lying away from the midline.

Ligament – Band of fibrous tissue that connects bone to bone.

Lumbar spine – Lower part of the back formed by lowest five non-fused vertebrae.

Malleolus – Rounded projection on either side of the ankle joint.

Manipulation – Moving with the hands.

Medial – Lying towards the midline.

Meniscus – Cushion of cartilage.

MET – Muscle energy technique.

Myofibrils – Small fibrils found in muscle tissue.

Neurone – Nerve cell.

NMT – Neuro muscular techniques.

Origin – Fixed end of attachment of muscle.

Osteoporosis – Abnormal brittleness of the bones.

Palpate – Examine by touch.

Pathology – Study of the causes, characteristics and effects of disease on the body.

Periosteum – Connective tissue covering bones.

Phalanges – Bones of fingers and toes.

Phlebitis – Inflammation of a vein.

Physiology – Study of the functions and actions of the body parts.

PNF – Proprioceptive neuromuscular facilitation.

Posterior – Back, behind.

Pronation – Turn downwards.

Proximal – Nearer to the trunk.

Quadriceps – Extensor muscles of the front of the thigh.

Referred pain – Pain felt on a body surface away from the pathological lesion.

Rotation – Turning round on an axis, external/lateral rotation, internal/medial rotation.

Skeletal muscle – Muscles which are attached to bone.

Smooth muscle – Involuntary muscle.

STR – Soft tissue release.

Supination – Turn face upwards.

Tendon – Fibrous tissue attaches skeletal muscle to bone.

Thoracic spine – Part of spine to which ribs attach, twelve vertebrae.

Thrombosis – Blood clot within a blood vessel.

Training cycle – Time devoted to specific exercise, interspersed with rest.

Varicose – Dilated.

Vasodilation – Increase in diameter of blood vessels.

Ventricle – Lower chambers of the heart.

Verruca – Growth in skin caused by virus, common on feet and infectious.

Wart – Hard growth on skin, caused by virus and can be infectious.

Index